Adrenal Glands - The Current Stage and New Perspectives of Diseases and Treatment

Edited by Diana Loreta Păun, Pasquale Cianci and Enrico Restini

Published in London, United Kingdom

Adrenal Glands - The Current Stage and New Perspectives of Diseases and Treatment
http://dx.doi.org/10.5772/intechopen.102209
Edited by Diana Loreta Păun, Pasquale Cianci and Enrico Restini

Contributors
Ali Gamal Ahmed Al-kaf, Ravi Kant Narayan, Ashutosh Kumar, Manika Verma, Ghemigian Mariana Adina, Dumitru Nicoleta, Aída Verónica Araya, Claudio Liberman, Claudia Munizaga, Pedro Pineda, Marcela Barberán, Francisco Cordero, Alejandra Lanas, Luis Toro, Monica Livia Gheorghiu, Sofia Maria Lider Burciulescu, Berta Carvalho, Filipa Carvalho, Davide Carvalho, Radu Mirica, Sorin Paun, Thawatchai Tullavardhana

First published in London, United Kingdom, 2024 by IntechOpen
IntechOpen is the global imprint of INTECHOPEN LIMITED, registered in England and Wales, registration number: 11086078, 5 Princes Gate Court, London, SW7 2QJ, United Kingdom

British Library Cataloguing-in-Publication Data
A catalogue record for this book is available from the British Library

Additional hard and PDF copies can be obtained from orders@intechopen.com

Adrenal Glands - The Current Stage and New Perspectives of Diseases and Treatment
Edited by Diana Loreta Păun, Pasquale Cianci and Enrico Restini
p. cm.
Print ISBN 978-1-80356-686-3
Online ISBN 978-1-80356-687-0
eBook (PDF) ISBN 978-1-80356-688-7

For EU product safety concerns:
IN TECH d.o.o., Prolaz Marije Krucifikse Kozulić 3, 51000 Rijeka, Croatia,
info@intechopen.com or visit our website at intechopen.com.

Meet the editors

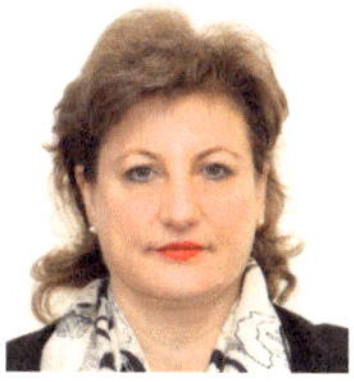

Diana Loreta Păun, MD, Ph.D., FACE, is an Associate Professor of Endocrinology at the University of Medicine and Pharmacy and an endocrinologist at the National Institute of Endocrinology, Bucharest, Romania. Dr. Paun has acquired a comprehensive array of qualifications within her field, encompassing diabetology, osteoporosis, endocrine ultrasonography, and public health. She was General Manager of the Institute of Endocrinology from 2006 to 2015. In 2019, she became the Presidential Advisor for Health to the president of Romania. Dr. Paun is a fellow of the American College of Endocrinology, former president of the Romanian chapter of the American Association of Clinical Endocrinologists (AACE), and a member of the Romanian Societies of Endocrinology and Psychoneuroendocrinology, and the Romanian Association of Clinical Endocrinologists.

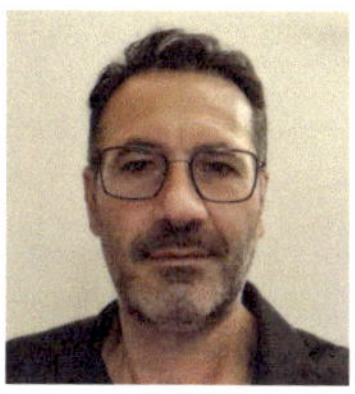

Pasquale Cianci is a general surgeon in the Department of Surgery and Traumatology, ASL BAT, Andria, Italy. He obtained a Ph.D. at the University of Foggia, Italy. He is a fellow of the American College of Surgeons (FACS). At the University of Foggia, Italy, he is a contract Professor of General and Emergency Surgery, Gastroenterology, and Human Physiology in the Nursing Science and Physiotherapy Courses. He is also a Professor of Surgical Anatomy at the same university's specialty school in general surgery. He is a member of several scientific surgical societies, including the European Association of Endoscopic Surgery (EAES), Italian Society of Endoscopic Surgery and New Technologies (SICE), Association of Italian Hospital Surgeons (ACOI), American College of Surgeons (ACS). He is the author of eighty national and international scientific papers, books, and book chapters. He is also an editorial board member of *Frontiers in Surgical Oncology, BMC Surgery*, and *Annals of Medicine*. He has served as faculty at numerous national and international surgical congresses. Dr. Cianci has a special interest in mini-invasive surgery, endocrine surgery, and coloproctology.

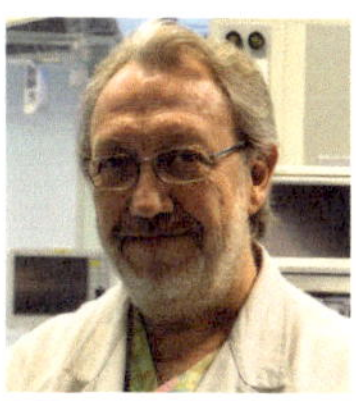

Enrico Restini is head of the Department of Surgery and Traumatology, ASL BAT, Andria, Italy. He is a contract Professor of Surgery and Health Management and an expert in advanced technologies and their impact on health organizations (i.e., Health Technology Assessment) at Libera Università Mediterranea (LUM), Baria, Italy. He is a member of the Society of American Gastrointestinal and Endoscopic Surgeons (SAGES), Italian Society of Endoscopic and New Technologies (SICE), Italian Society of Bariatric Surgery (SICOB), SIC, Italian Society of Private Hospital Surgery, and Association of Italian Hospital Surgeons (ACOI). He is a founding member of the Foundation for Research on Integrative Oncological Therapies (ARTOI), and he has been a SICE National Councilor since 2012. He has served as faculty at numerous national and international surgical congresses and is the author of fifty national and international scientific papers. His special interests include laparoscopic surgery, robotic surgery, endocrine surgery, digestive surgery, and oncological surgery.

Contents

Preface

In the context of the accelerated progress in endocrinology, addressing adrenal gland pathology and the latest therapeutic developments in adrenal diseases presents a significant challenge.

The adrenal gland is essential for survival and represents the primary endocrine pathway for adapting to stress, making its pathology complex and with profound implications for the entire body.

This book delves into the anatomy, physiology, and pathology of the adrenal glands, striving to present the current state of knowledge in the field and new therapeutic perspectives.

The first section of the book is dedicated to describing the embryology, anatomy, and physiology of the adrenal glands, with a separate chapter detailing the hormones secreted by the adrenals and their effects on the body.

The second section of the book extensively covers adrenal diseases with clinical significance. From Cushing's syndrome to primary aldosteronism, from congenital adrenal hyperplasia to pheochromocytoma, each chapter in this section is like a standalone volume, exploring diagnostic and therapeutic aspects that can be reviewed and redefined, presented in detail, and complemented with new data.

Equally important are the interconnections that the adrenal gland has within the human body, laying the groundwork for describing the intimate mechanisms that lead to adrenal diseases affecting other tissues and organs, as well as strategic considerations regarding treatment. Surgical treatment is discussed separately, given the complexity of this therapy and the technical advancements accumulated in recent years.

This book, addressing both practicing endocrinologists and specialists from other medical fields, explores the mysteries of adrenal diseases and provides a comprehensive overview of the current state of knowledge about this gland. It offers an easy-to-follow format that focuses on the most significant advancements in the etiopathogenesis, clinical and laboratory diagnosis, and treatment of these conditions.

I would like to express my gratitude to all the chapter authors for their courage in addressing this complex and fascinating pathology and for their support in this endeavor.

Diana Loreta Păun
Department of Endocrinology,
"Carol Davila" University of Medicine and Pharmacy,
Bucharest, Romania

Pasquale Cianci and Enrico Restini
"Lorenzo Bonomo" Hospital-ASL BAT,
Department of Surgery and Traumatology,
Andria (Puglia), Italy

Section 1

Anatomy and Physiology of the Adrenal Glands

Chapter 1

The Development and Anatomy of Adrenal Glands

Ravi Kant Narayan, Ashutosh Kumar and Manika Verma

Abstract

The retroperitoneal adrenals are situated in the epigastric region of the abdomen, on the upper pole of either kidney. The glands are golden-yellow in color. The right adrenal is triangular or pyramidal, and the left one is semi-circular or crescentic in shape. The blood supply rate per gram of tissue for the adrenal gland is one of the highest. The two parts of the gland are derived from two different embryological tissues. This chapter discusses the normal macro- and microscopic anatomy of the gland along with its embryological development.

Keywords: adrenal, glands, retroperitoneal, microscopic anatomy, embryology

1. Introduction

The kidneys' fibrous capsule (renal fascia) wraps a wedged glandular and neuroendocrine tissue to its upper pole. These tissue masses are referred to as adrenal glands [1]. The adrenal glands were initially described in detail by Italian anatomist Bartolomeo Eustachi in 1563–1564. Adrenal is a Latin word where "*ad*" means "near", and "*ren*" means "kidney". The paired structure was termed "suprarenal", another Latin word where "*supra*" means "above", by Jean Riolan the Younger in 1629 [2]. These are endocrine glands, therefore, receive profuse blood supply via multiple arteries. In gross appearance, these are yellowish [3].

Adrenal glands have two major parts: the cortex and the medulla. These two parts share the similarity in their location, apart from which they differ in their ontogeny, phylogeny, architecture, and function [4]. In this chapter, the adrenals are discussed under the following headings:

1. Location, external features, & coverings

2. Gross appearance and microscopic architecture

3. Arterial supply, Venous & Lymphatic drainage

4. Nerve innervations

5. Development

2. Location, external features, & coverings

The retroperitoneal adrenals are situated in the epigastric region of the abdomen, on the upper pole of either kidney (**Figure 1**). The right adrenal being pyramidal in shape, has an apex, a base, two surfaces (anterior and posterior), and three borders (medial and

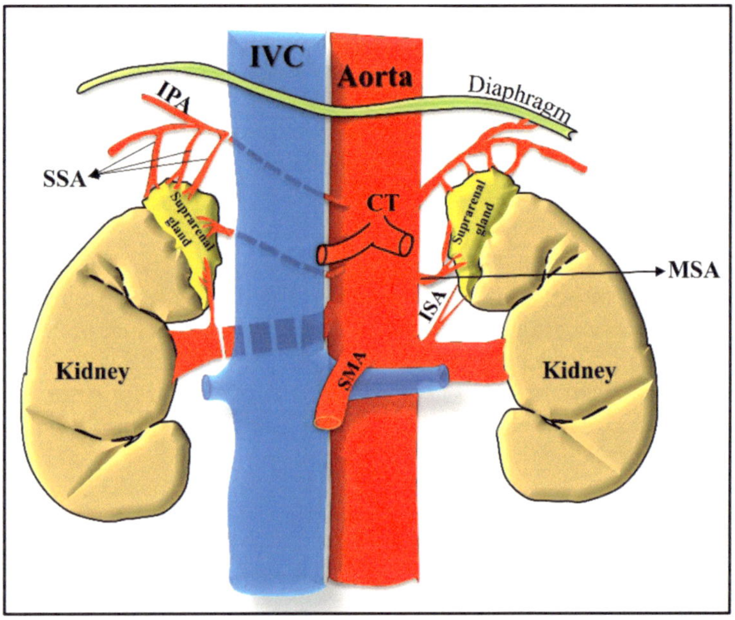

Figure 1.
Illustration of the adrenal/ suprarenal gland's location on the upper pole of both kidneys and the blood supply of the glands (IVC – inferior vena cava, IPA – inferior phrenic artery, CT – coeliac trunk, SMA – superior mesenteric artery, SSA – superior suprarenal artery, MSA – middle suprarenal artery, ISA – inferior suprarenal artery).

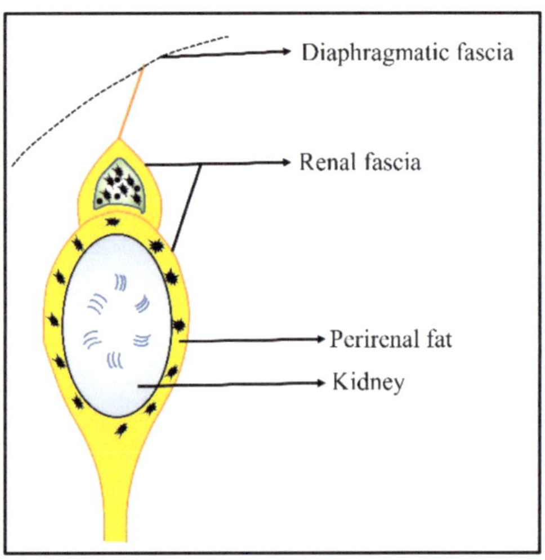

Figure 2.
Sectional illustration of the renal fascia enveloping the kidney, and adrenal gland, extending to fuse with the diaphragmatic fascia.

lateral) [4]. The posteromedial surface is related to the diaphragm, and the inferior vena cava is on the anteromedial surface. Different aspects of the liver are related to the right adrenal; the right lobe of the liver lies anteriorly, while the bare area is located superior to the gland. The right kidney's upper pole is inferolateral to the endocrine structure. The crescentic left adrenal has two ends (narrow upper end and rounded lower end), two borders (medial and lateral), and two surfaces (anterior and posterior). The stomach lies anteriorly, the diaphragm posteromedially, and the kidney inferolateral [1].

The adrenals are surrounded by two sheaths, a layer of loose areolar tissue directly encapsulating the glands, and is composed of a significant quantity of fat. At the same time, the outer layer is the continuation of renal fascia, which also forms a thin septum separating the kidney from the adrenal above. An extension of the fascia connects the adrenal capsule's outer layer to the diaphragm's underlying peritoneal layer, which is attributed to the movement of the gland during respiration (**Figure 2**) [5].

3. Gross appearance and microscopic architecture

The size of the adrenal glands is around 5 cm long, 3 cm wide, and up to 1 cm thick. They weigh about 7 and 10 grams together in an adult person. The glands are golden-yellow in color (**Figure 3**) [3]. The right adrenal is triangular or pyramidal, and the left one is semi-circular or crescentic in shape. The external yellow-gold adrenal cortex and the inner brown-red adrenal medulla could easily be demarcated by gross examination of the cut surface of the adrenal gland [1, 6].

Microscopically, the adrenal cortex can be divided into three separate zones depending upon the arrangement of the cells (**Figure 4**). These are zona glomerulosa, zona fasciculata and zona reticularis. Each zone produces specific hormones pouring into the sinusoids running between the cells [7].

3.1 Zona glomerulosa

This is the outermost zone of the cortex, located just underneath the fibrous capsule. The cells are arranged in oval clusters giving the term "glomerulosa". Aldosterone

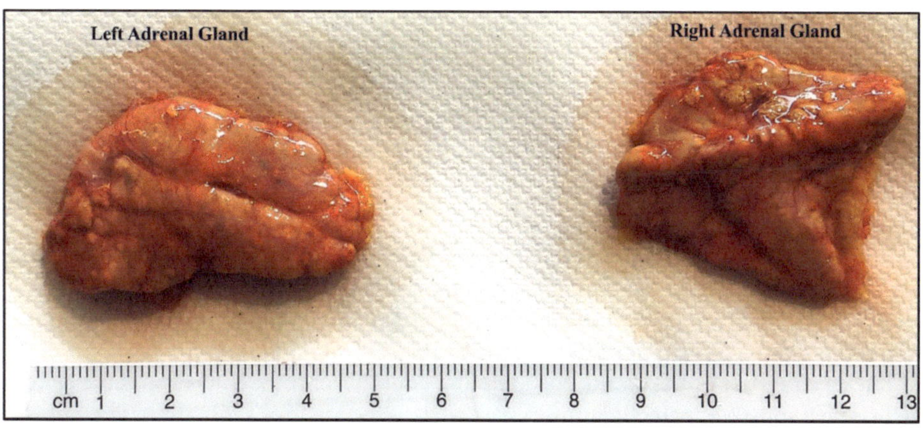

Figure 3.
Image of adrenal glands, anterior (left) and posterior (right) surface, with scale for measuring length. Image courtesy: Mikael Häggström, MD. Public Domain (CC0 1.0).

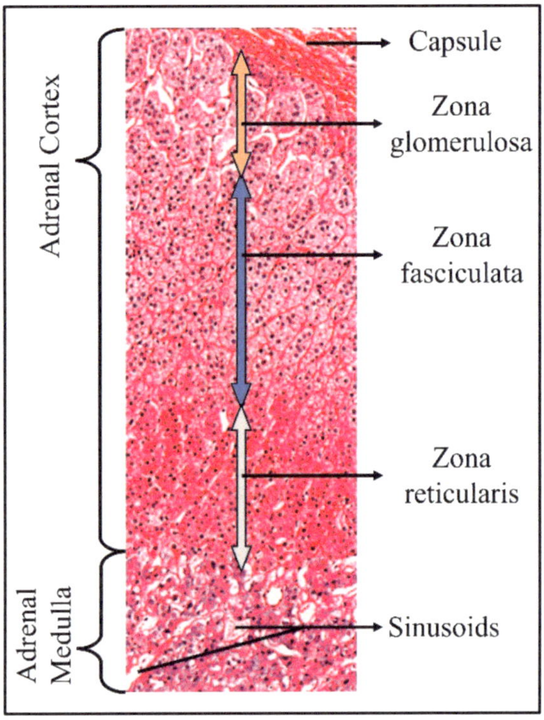

Figure 4.
Histological image of the adrenal showing different zones of the cortex and the medulla.

synthase, an enzyme, works primarily in this layer to produce the mineralocorticoid aldosterone, which is crucial for controlling blood pressure and maintaining salt concentration (**Table 1**) [5].

3.2 Zona fasciculata

The cells in this zone are organized in columns, or tape-like arrangements (hence the term 'fasciculata') radially orientated toward the medulla. It makes up around 80% of the cortex's volume, making it the thickest of the three layers. The fasciculata cells release glucocorticoids like cortisol, which regulates the metabolism of proteins, fats, and sugars (**Table 1**) [5].

3.3 Zona reticularis

The innermost layer of the adrenal cortex lies adjacent to the medulla. Here the tiny cells are arranged in the form of irregular cords and clusters (hence the term 'reticularis'). The capillaries and connective tissue can be found between these cords. These cells produce androgens in humans (**Table 1**) [5].

The central part of the gland, the medulla, contains chromaffin cells. These cells are the primary source of catecholamines, i.e., adrenaline and noradrenaline. The fight-or-flight response is characterized by the effects of the catecholamines, which include elevated heart rate and blood pressure, constriction of blood vessels in the skin and

Zones of the Adrenal gland	Hormones secreted	Hormonal effects	Regulatory controls
Zona Glomerulosa	Mineralocorticoids, Aldosterone	Increases renal reabsorption of sodium and water. It also increases urinary loss of potassium.	Mineralocorticoid secretion is stimulated by the activation of the renin-angiotensin system and is inhibited by hormones opposing that system.
Zona Fasciculata	Glucocorticoids, Cortisol	Glucocorticoids increase rates of glucose and glycogen formation by the liver.	Glucocorticoids secretion is stimulated by the Adrenocorticotropic hormone (ACTH)
Zona Reticularis	Androgens	Stimulates the development of pubic hair in boys and girls before puberty	Androgen secretion is stimulated by ACTH
Adrenal Medulla	Adrenaline And Noradrenaline	Increases cardiac activity, blood pressure, glycogen breakdown, and blood glucose levels.	Adrenaline and Noradrenaline secretion are stimulated by sympathetic preganglionic fibers during sympathetic activation.

Table 1.
Secretions of adrenal gland zones, their effects, and their regulatory controls.

gastrointestinal tract, dilatation of smooth muscle (bronchioles and capillaries), and increased metabolism (**Table 1**) [5].

4. Arterial supply, venous & lymphatic drainage

The blood supply rate per gram of tissue for the adrenal gland is one of the highest. This could only be achieved due to several arterial branches entering the gland, which are derived from three major branches (**Figure 1**) [8–10]:

a. Superior suprarenal artery - a branch of the inferior phrenic artery

b. Middle suprarenal artery - a direct branch of the abdominal aorta

c. Inferior suprarenal artery - a branch of the renal artery

On the contrary, each gland is drained by a single vein, namely

a. Right suprarenal vein which drains directly into the inferior vena cava

b. Left suprarenal vein which drains into the left renal or inferior phrenic vein.

The short cortical arteries form the subcapsular plexus branches. The plexus then provides an anastomosing network of capillary sinusoids that constitute the cortex's vascular system. These sinusoids infiltrate between the cords of zona fasciculata and then create the deep plexus in the zona reticularis, where they drain into minute venules that confluence with the principal vein of the medulla [7].

The medulla receives blood from two sources, the arterial medullary arterioles and the venous cortical sinusoidal capillaries, which have already fed the cortex and are high in adrenocorticosteroids. Long cortical arteries drop through the cortex from the subcapsular plexus and ramify into a dense network of dilated capillaries around the medullary secretory cells. The medullary capillaries then drain into the central medullary vein. Subsequently, the venous drainage of the cortex also supplies the medullary cells while crossing through the medulla on their way to the central medullary vein. The corticosteroids in the cortical venules are thought to significantly impact the medulla's ability to synthesize adrenaline [5, 7].

The lymph from the paired glands drains into lateral aortic nodes. The lymphatic vessels have been observed in the capsule, the connective tissue around the larger blood vessels, and the parenchyma of the adrenal medulla [11].

5. Nerve innervations

The adrenal is a neuroendocrine gland, i.e., the gland is regulated by both the pituitary hormones and nerve innervations. The cortical part of the gland is under the regulation of adrenocorticotrophic hormone released by the anterior lobe of the pituitary [5].

The adrenal medulla is considered a modified sympathetic ganglion as it is innervated by the myelinated pre-ganglionic sympathetic fibers coming from T5–T11 (splanchnic nerves) spinal levels and pours its secretion into the sinusoids, unlike other sympathetic ganglions [5].

6. Development

Either part of the adrenal gland is derived from two different embryological tissues. The adrenal cortex is derived from proliferated mesothelial cells around 5–6 weeks post-conception, while the medulla originates from the neural crest (**Figure 5**). The foetal adrenal cortex surrounds the growing adrenal medulla, and the entire gland is enclosed in a mesodermal layer that isolates it from the nearby developing gonad and kidney. The foetal adrenal cortex separates into two histologically distinct zones at about 9 weeks gestation: the definitive and foetal zones. Between the definitive and foetal zones, a third layer, the transitional zone, develops in the third trimester. The zona glomerulosa, the adrenal cortex's outer layer that generates mineralocorticoids, and the zona fasciculata, which produces glucocorticoids, are formed by 6 months of age from the definitive and transitional zones. The foetal cortex involutes throughout the first year of life, and the zona reticularis, which generates androgens, develops as the adrenal cortex's innermost layer. By 3 to 4 years, the zona reticularis differentiates into a separate layer (**Figure 6**) [6, 12].

It is interesting to note that medullary and cortical tissues combine to form a single organ in mammals, whereas they form into two separate organs in pre-vertebrates. The migration of medullary cells into the cortex, which starts in the seventh week of

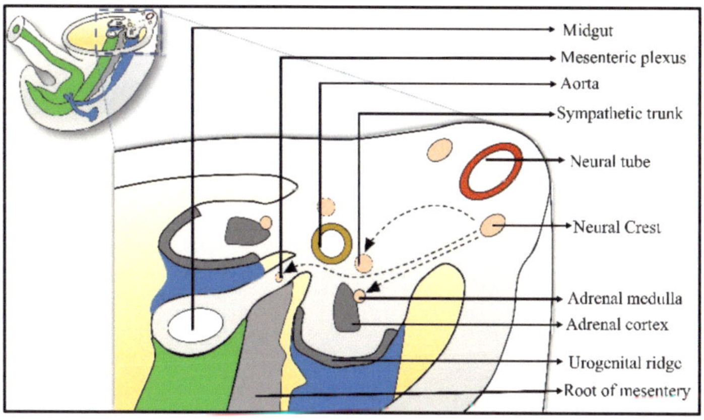

Figure 5.
Illustration of magnified view of a foetal section showing the developmental tissues of the adrenal cortex and medulla.

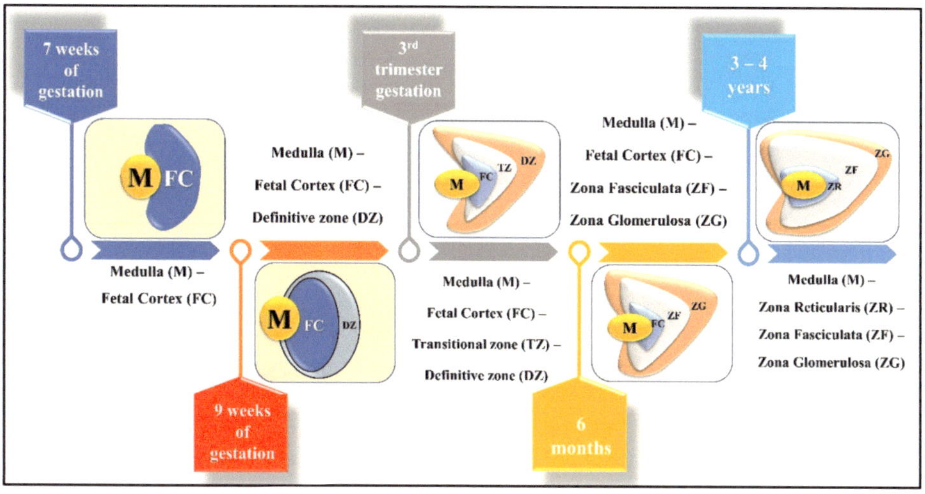

Figure 6.
Illustration of the timeline for the development of the zones of the adrenal cortex and the medulla in a foetus.

pregnancy, allows the primitive medullary and cortical cells to unite to form the adrenal gland. By the second trimester, the foetal adrenal cortex surrounds the medulla, and the entire gland is encased by a mesodermal layer, which isolates the adrenal glands from the nearby retroperitoneal structures [6, 13, 14].

Author details

Ravi Kant Narayan[1*], Ashutosh Kumar[2] and Manika Verma[3]

1 Dr.B.C. Roy Multi Speciality Medical Research Centre, IIT Kharagpur, India

2 All India Institute of Medical Sciences, Patna, India

3 Rajendra Institute of Medical Sciences, Ranchi, India

*Address all correspondence to: narayanintouch@gmail.com

References

[1] Standring S. Kidney and ureter. In: Gray's Anatomy [Internet]. 41st ed. London: Elsevier; 2016. [cited 2022 Sep 23] p. 1239-1240. Available from: https://www.elsevier.com/books/grays-anatomy/standring/978-0-7020-7705-0

[2] Schmidt JE. Medical discoveries: Who and when: A dictionary listing thousands of medical and related scientific discoveries in alphabetical order, giving in each case the name of the discoverer, his profession, nationality, and floruit, and the date of the discovery. Springfield (Ill.): Charles C. Thomas; 1959. p. 555

[3] Neville AM, O'Hare MJ. The Human Adrenal Cortex [Internet]. 1st ed. London: Springer London; 1982 [cited 2022 Sep 23]. Available from: http://link.springer.com/10.1007/978-1-4471-1317-1

[4] Kidneys SV. Ureters, and Suprarenal Glands. In: Textbook of Anatomy: Abdomen and Lower Limb. 2nd ed. New Delhi: Elsevier India; 2014. pp. 180-181

[5] Moore KL, Dalley AF, Agur AMR. Clinically Oriented Anatomy. Philadelphia: Lippincott Williams & Wilkins; 2013. p. 1171

[6] Vasudevan S, Brandt ML. Adrenal gland embryology, anatomy, and physiology. In: Ledbetter DJ, Johnson PRV, editors. Endocrine Surgery in Children [Internet]. Berlin, Heidelberg: Springer; 2018 [cited 2022 Sep 23]. pp. 77-85. DOI: 10.1007/978-3-662-54256-9_7

[7] Young B, Woodford P, O'Dowd G. Adrenal glands. In: Wheater's Functional Histology: A Text and Colour Atlas. 6th ed. London, England: Churchill Livingstone; 2013. pp. 328-321

[8] Narayan RK, Asghar A, Ghosh SK, Bharti S. Adrenal myelolipoma mimics ectopic adrenal or renal tissue: An incidental finding during cadaveric dissection. Acta Endocrinol Buchar Rom. 2021;**17**(1):111-116

[9] Priya A, Narayan R, Ghosh S. Prevalence and clinical relevance of the anatomical variations of suprarenal arteries: A review. Anatomy & Cell Biology. 2022;**55**(1):28-39. DOI: 10.5115/acb.21.211

[10] Priya A, Narayan R, Ghosh S. Unilateral variations of inferior phrenic and suprarenal arteries: A case study with commentary on its clinical importance. Translational Research in Anatomy. 1 Nov 2021;**25**:100147. DOI: 10.1016/j.tria.2021.100147

[11] Ross M, Pawlina W. Endocrine organs. In: Histology: A Text and Atlas. 7th ed. London: Wolters Kluwer Health; 2016. pp. 767-768

[12] Mitty HA. Embryology, anatomy, and anomalies of the adrenal gland. Seminars in Roentgenology. 1988;**23**(4):271-279

[13] Avisse C, Marcus C, Patey M, Ladam-Marcus V, Delattre JF, Flament JB. Surgical anatomy and embryology of the adrenal glands. The Surgical Clinics of North America. 2000;**80**(1):403-415

[14] Barwick TD, Malhotra A, Webb JAW, Savage MO, Reznek RH. Embryology of the adrenal glands and its relevance to diagnostic imaging. Clinical Radiology. 2005;**60**(9):953-959

Chapter 2

Adrenal Cortex Hormones

Ali Gamal Ahmed Al-kaf

Abstract

Over 50 different steroids, including precursors to other steroid hormones, are secreted by the adrenal glands, which are located directly above the kidneys. Aldosterone and hydrocortisone, however, are the two most significant hormonal steroids created by the adrenal cortex. Since aldosterone is too expensive to produce commercially, other semi-synthetic analogues are now used to treat Addison's disease in its place. Fludrocortisone, for example, greatly increases both salt retention and anti-inflammatory activity when combined with hydrocortisone. The kidneys' ability to reabsorb sodium is increased by aldosterone. Increased blood volume will follow an increase in plasma sodium concentration. Additionally, aldosterone boosts potassium ion excretion. Addison's disease is brought on by inconsistency. Glycogen storage synthesis is induced by the synthesis of glycogen synthase, and gluconeogenesis (the production of glucose from glucose) is induced in the liver.

Keywords: steroid hormones, adrenal glands, synthesis, metabolism, structure-activity relationship, mechanism and activity

1. Introduction

Over 50 different steroids, including precursors to other steroid hormones, are secreted by the adrenal glands, which are located directly above the kidneys. Aldosterone and hydrocortisone, however, which are the most significant hormonal steroids produced by the adrenal cortex, are only used to treat Addison's disease [1]. An 11-OH and an 18-CHO in the naturally occurring hormone aldosterone naturally bridge to form a hemiacetal.

Because aldosterone is too expensive to produce commercially, other semi-synthetic analogues are now used to treat Addison's disease instead [1].

Fludrocortisone, for example, greatly increases both salt retention and anti-inflammatory activity when added to hydrocortisone [2, 3].

They also secrete a number of vital hormones that are crucial for maintaining a healthy immune system, metabolic rate, and salt and water balance in the body (**Tables 1–5**).

IntechOpen

Group of hormones	Double bond	Substitutes		
		X_1	X_2	R
Corticosteroids	en-4 Dien- 1,4	=O	-H -OH =O	H_2C—OH C=O -----OH
Gestogens	en-4	=O	-H	CH_3 C=O
Androgens	en-4	=O	-H	-OH
Estrogens	Trien-1,3,5 (No C-19)	-OH	-H	-OH =O

Table 1.
Chemical structure of steroid hormones [3].

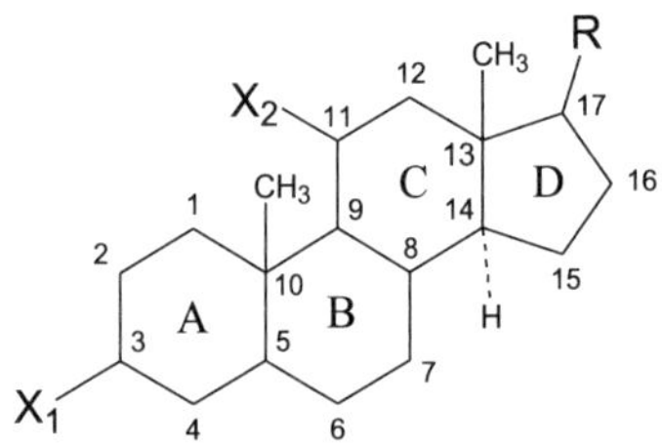

Medicinal substances	Color of solution	Florescence
Dezoxycortone acetate	Yellow (after addition of water becomes violet)	Green-yellow color with red florescence (after addition of ethanol)
Cortisone acetate	Red (after heating to 80–90°C becomes orange) "within 2 minutes"	Yellow (within 5 minutes under UV lamp)
Hydrocortisone	Yellow transferred into red (within 5 minutes)	Yellow green transferred into green (after addition of water)
Prednisolone	Green transferred into red	Not available (absent)

Table 2.
Results of the reaction between corticosteroids with conc. H_2SO_4 [3–5].

Medicinal substances	Solvent	Max. absorption (nm)	Refractive index
Dezoxy cortone acetate	Ethanol	241	430–450
Cortisone acetate	Ethanol	238	390
Hydrocortisone acetate	Ethanol	241	395
Prednisolone	Methanol	242	400–430

Table 3.
Conditions of spectrophotometric determination of corticosteroids [3–5].

Clinical antirheumatic enhancement factors			
Functional group	**Factor**	**Functional group**	**Factor**
1-Dehydro	2.8	16 α-Methyl	1.6
6-Dehydro	0.9	6 β-Methyl	1.3
6 α-Methyl	0.9	16 α, 17 α-Isopropylidenedioxy	0.6
6 α-Fluoro	1.9	17 α-Acetoxy	0.3
9 α-Fluoro	4.9	21-Deoxy	0.2
16 α-Hydroxy	0.3	21-Methyl	0.3

Table 4.
Effects of substituents on glucocorticoid activity.

Functional group	Glycogen deposition	Anti-inflammatory activity	Effects on urinary sodium
9 α-Fluoro	10	7–10	+ + +
9 α-Chloro	3–5	3	+ +
9 α-Bromo	0.4		+
12 α-Fluoro	6–8		+ +
12 α-Chloro	4		
1-Dehydro	3–4	3–4	—
6-Dehydro	0.5–0.7		+
2 α-Methyl	3–6	1–4	+ +
6 α-Methyl	2–3	1–2	—
16 α-Hydroxy	0.4–0.5	0.1–0.2	—
17 α-Hydroxy	1–2	4	—

Table 5.
Enhancement factors for various functional groups of corticosteroids.

2. Chemistry of steroid hormones

The general formula for the basic structure of the steroid compounds may be represented as follows [3].

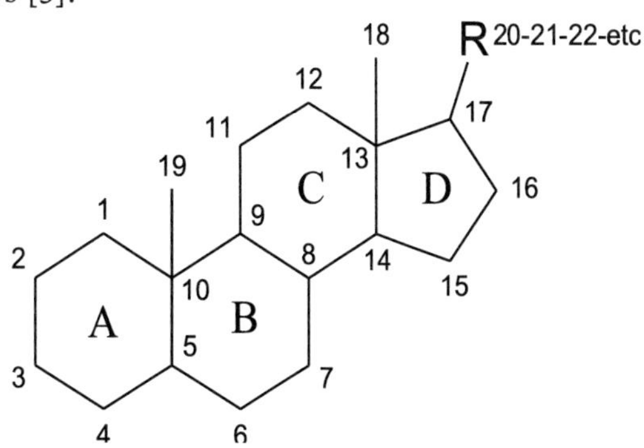

2.1 General steroid formula

In 1956, N.N. Suvoroviy with his colleagues (Allunion Scientific Research of Chemical and Physical Institute) were shown the ability of obtaining cortisone from solasodine from the plant *Solanum* [3, 4].

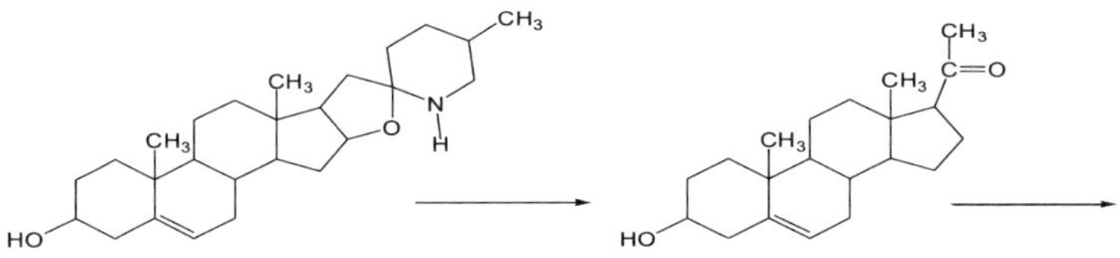

Solasodine Pregnenolone

aviculare, family of *Solanaceae*.

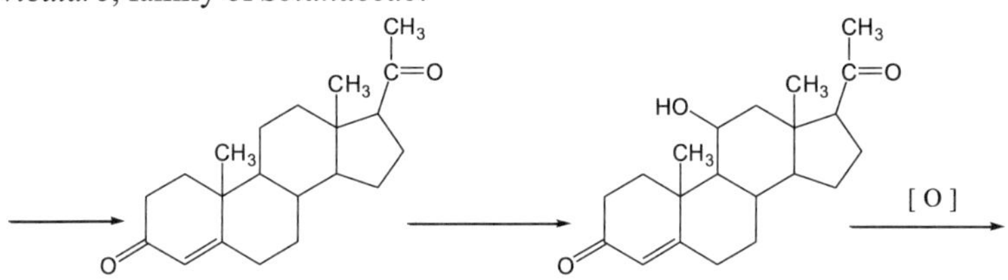

Progesterone 11- α -oxy progesterone

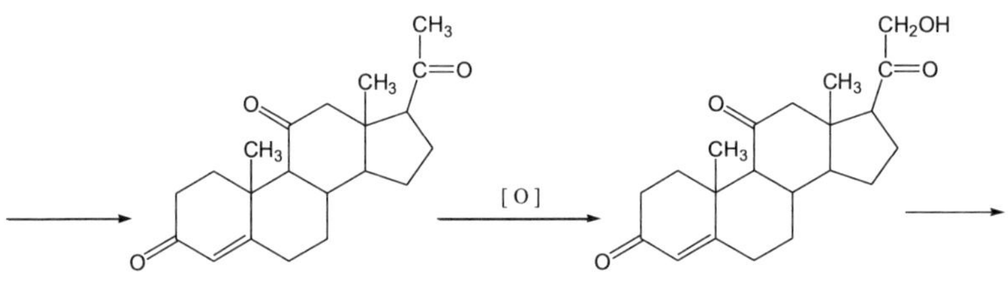

11- dihydrocorticosterone

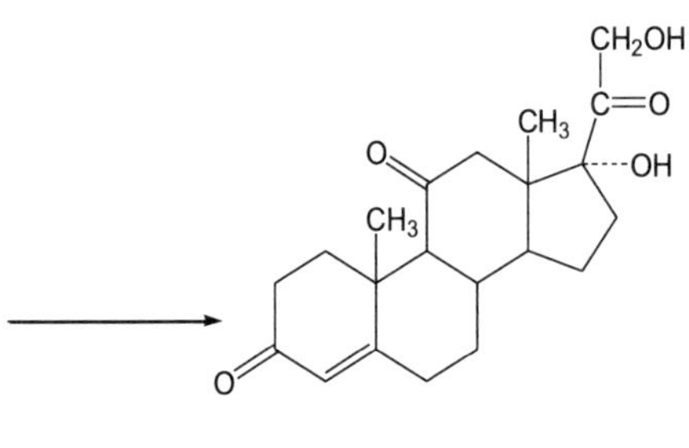

Cortisone

Corticosteroids may be differentiated from each other by reaction on this or other functional groups [3].

By heating on water bath, spiritus solutions of corticosteroids with phenylhydrazine solution formed yellow color. This reaction occurred with ketonic group, for example [3].

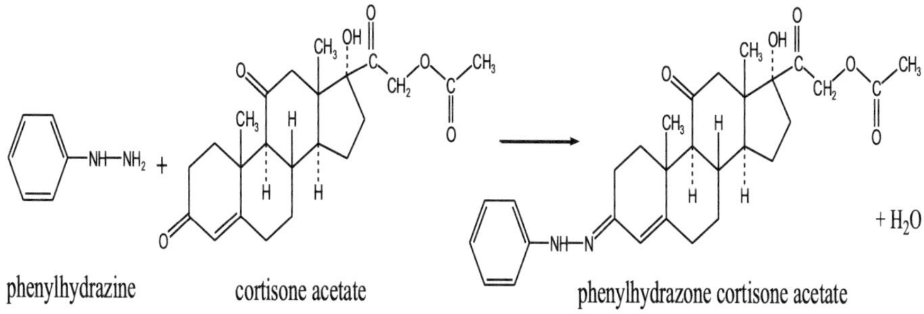

Reaction for obtaining acetohydroxamic acid which reacts with iron salts (III) formed compounds colored in dark cherry (cortisone acetate) or red-brown color (dezoxycortone acetate) [3].

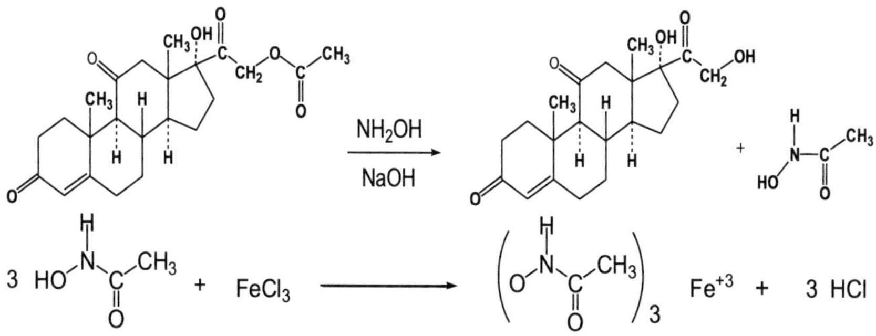

Acetyl group may be detected after hydrolysis of cortisone and hydrocortisone acetate in spiritus solution of hydroxid potassium and subsequent addition of conc. Sulfuric acid which forms ethyl acetate with characteristic odor. For identification of hydrocortisone acetate: [3].

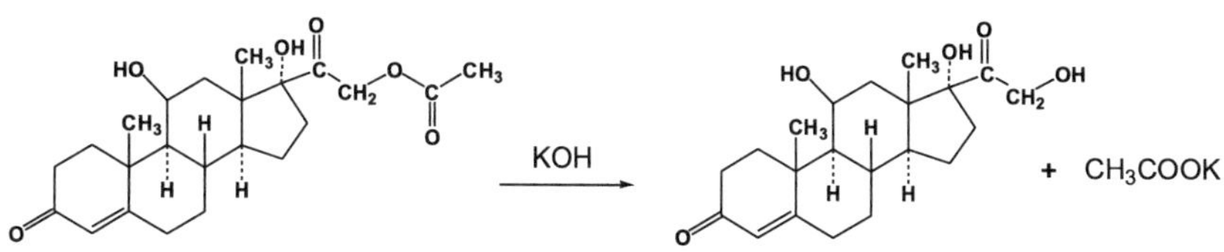

$$2\,CH_3COOK + H_2SO_4 + 2\,C_2H_5OH \longrightarrow 2CH_3COOC_2H_5 + K_2SO_4 + 2\,H_2O$$

The adrenal glands (which lie just above the kidneys) secrete over 50 different steroids, including precursors to other steroid hormones. However the most important hormonal steroids produced by the adrenal cortex are aldosterone and hydrocortisone [6–11].

2.2 Mineralocorticoids

They are used only for treatment of Addison's disease. The naturally occurring hormone aldosterone has an 11 β-OH and an 18-CHO that naturally bridge to form a hemiacetal [7–13].

Aldosterone is too expensive to produce commercially; therefore other semisynthetic analogues have taken its place for treatment of Addison's disease [12].

Adding a 9 α-halogen to hydrocortisone (e.g. Fludrocortisone) greatly increases both salt retention and anti-inflammatory activity [2, 3].

1- Mineralcorticoids (High Salt Retention)

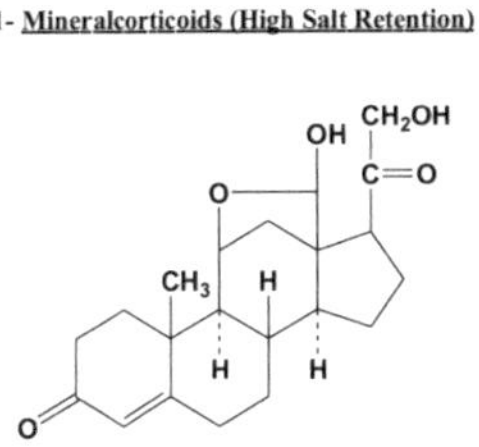

Aldosterone
(not commercially available)

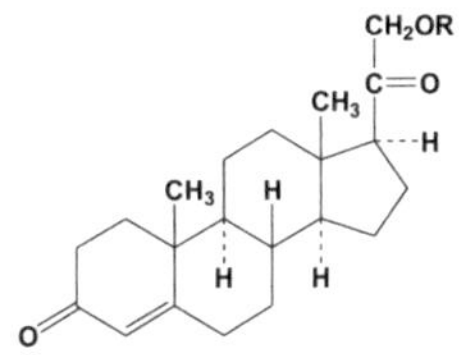

Deoxycorticosterone (R = H)

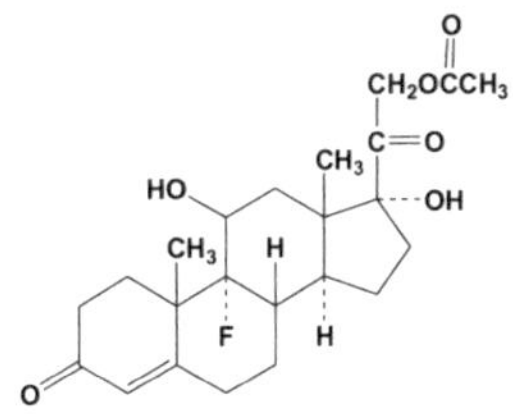

Fludrocortisone Acetate

Esters available:
Deoxycorticosterone Acetate: R = $COCH_3$
Deoxycorticosterone Pivalate: R = $COC(CH_3)_3$

The following table summarizes the relative effect of various substituents on salt retention and glucocorticoid activity. The salt-retaining actions are approximately additive. For example, a 9 α-fluoro group's + + + increase in salt retention can be eliminated by 6 α-methyl's - - - [2, 14–16].

2.3 Glucocorticoids with moderate to low salt retention

The glucocorticoids with moderate to low retention include cortisone, hydrocortisone, and their 1-enes prednisolone and prednisone [2, 14–16].

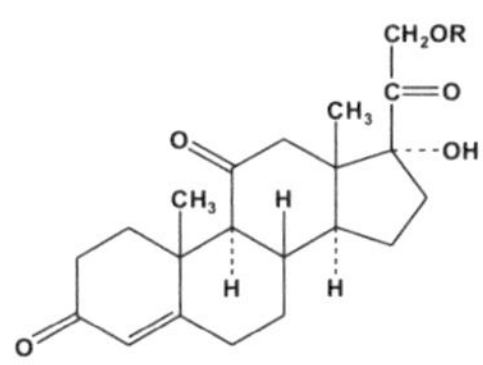

Cortisone (R = H)

Ester available:
Cortisone Acetate: R = $COCH_3$

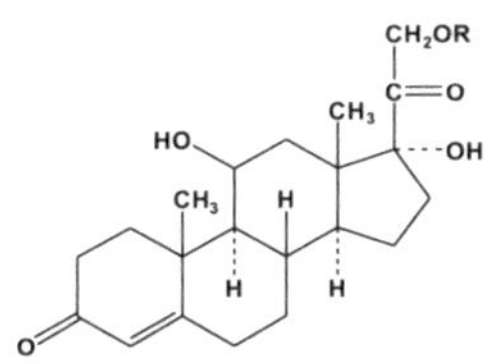

Hydrocortisone (R = H)
(or Cortisol)

Esters Available:
Hydrocortisone Acetate: R = $COCH_3$
Hydrocortisone Cypionate: R = $COCH_2CH_2$–cyclopentyl

Salts Available:
Hydrocortisone Sodium Phosphate: R = $PO_3^{=}(Na^+)_2$
Hydrocortisone Sodium Succinate:
R = $COCH_2CH_2COO^-Na^+$

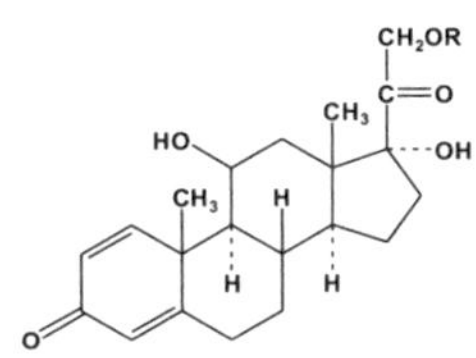

Prednisolone (R = H)

Salts Available:
Prednisolone Sodium Phosphate: R = $PO_3^{=}(Na^+)_2$
Prednisolone Sodium Succinate: R = $COCH_2CH_2COO^-Na^+$

Esters Available:
Prednisolone Acetate: R= Ac
Prednisolone Succinate: R = $COCH_2CH_2COOH$
Prednisolone Tebutate: R = $COCH_2C(CH_3)_3$

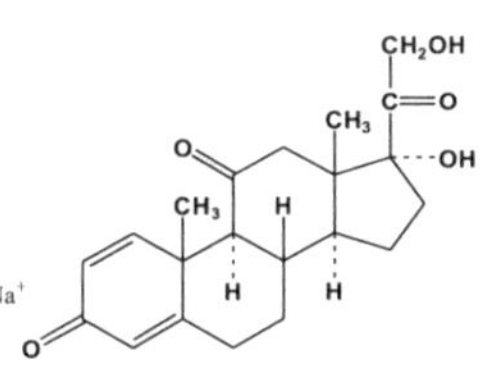

Prednisone

Fig... Natural and semisynthetic adrenal cortex hormones

An 11-OH maintains good topical anti-inflammatory activity, but 11-ones have little or none [2, 3, 14–16].

The 1-ene of prednisolone and prednisone increases anti-inflammatory activity by about a factor of 4 and somewhat decreases salt retention [2, 3, 14–16] (**Figures 1–13**).

The 11 β-OH of hydrocortisone is believed to be of major importance in binding to the receptors. Cortisone may be reduced in vivo to yield hydrocortisone as the active agent [2, 3, 14–16, 19–22].

Introduction of fluoro (F) to C6α and C9α positions increase both mineralocorticoid and glucocorticoid activity due to the electron-withdrawing inductive effect on the 11β-OH making it more acidic, therefore, better able to form noncovalent bonds with the receptor. A 9α-halo substituent also reduces oxidation of the 11 β-OH to the less active 11-one [2, 3, 14–16, 19–22].

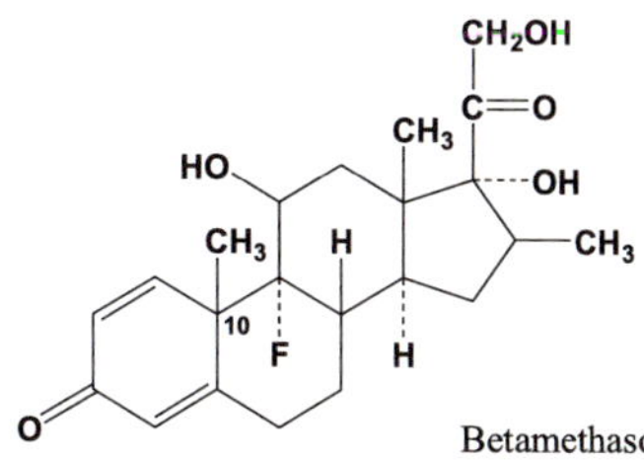

Betamethasone
(C10 β- methyl)

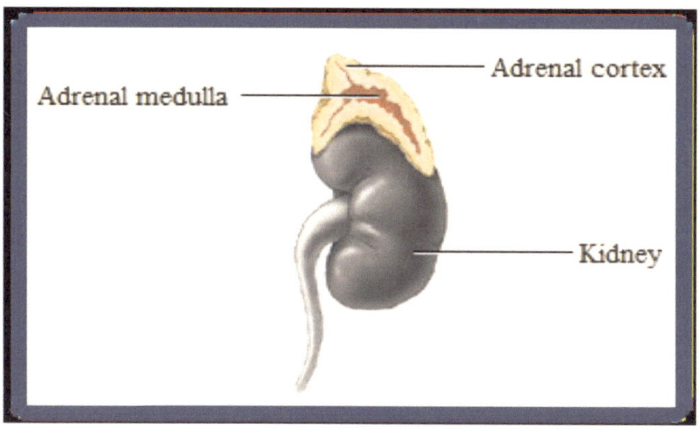

Figure 1.
Structure of adrenal gland.

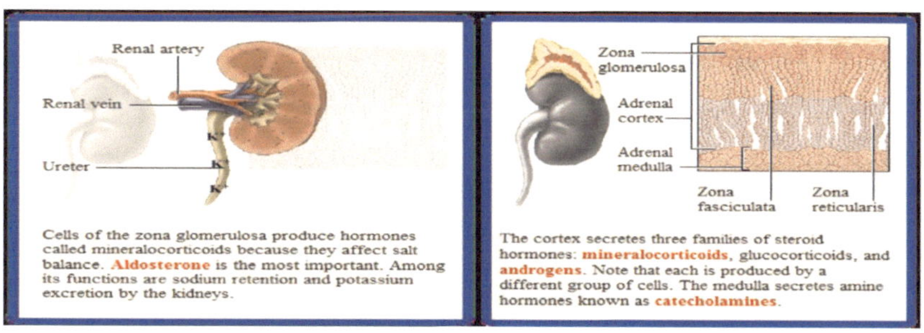

Figure 2.
(Left) Cells of the zona glomerulosa produce hormones called mineralocorticoids because they affect salt balance. ***Aldosterone*** *is the most important. Among its functions are sodium retention and potassium excretion by the kidneys. (Right) The cortex secretes three families of steroid hormones:* ***mineralocorticoids****, glucocorticoids, and* ***androgens****. Note that each is produced by a different group of cells. The medulla secretes amine hormones known as* ***catecholamines****.*

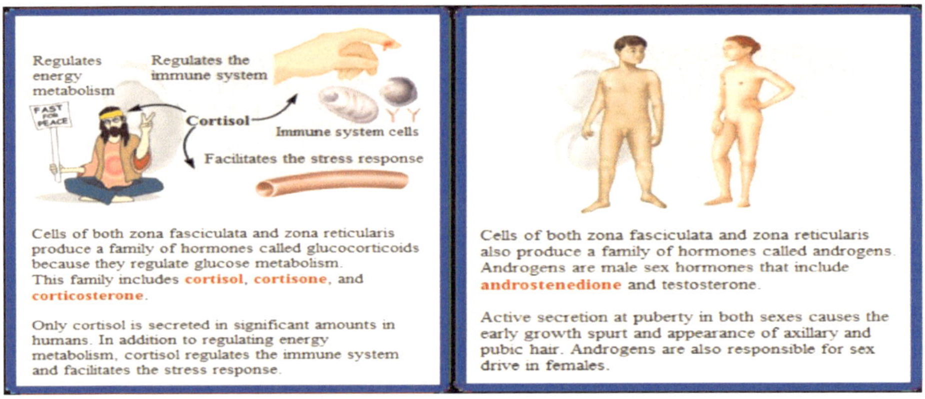

Figure 3.
(Left) Cells of both zona fasciculata and zona reticularis produce a family of hormones called glucocorticoids because they regulate glucose metabolism. This family includes ***cortisol, cortisone****, and* ***corticosterone****. Only cortisol is secreted in significant amounts in humans. In addition to regulating energy metabolism, cortisol regulates the immune system and facilitates the stress response. (Right) Cells of both zona fasciculate and zona reticularis also produce a family of hormones called androgens. Androgens are male sex hormones that include* ***androstenedione*** *and testosterone. Active secretion at puberty in both sexes causes the early growth spurt and appearance of axillary and pubic hair. Androgens are also responsible for sex drive in females.*

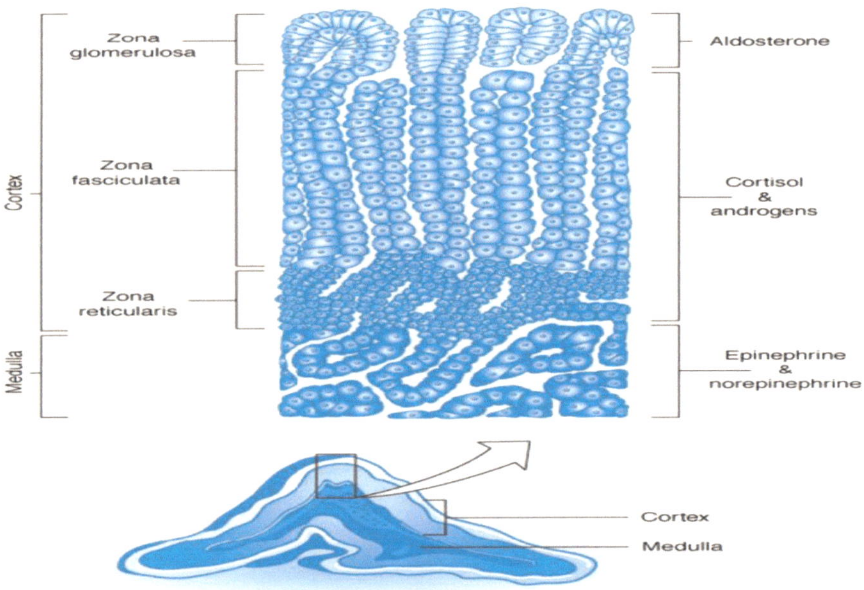

Figure 4.
Functional anatomy and zonation.

2.4 Glucocorticoids with very little or no salt retention

They include 16 α-hydroxy (Triamcinolone); 16 α-, 17 α-ketal; (Amcinolone, Desonide, Flunisolide, Triamcinolone acetonide, Flucinolone acetonide, Flurandrenolide) [2, 14–16, 23].

DOI: http://dx.doi.org/10.5772/intechopen.106785

Common Name	Previous Form	Current Form	Gene
Cholesterol side-chain cleavage enzyme	$P450_{SCC}$	CYP11A1	*CYP11A1*
3β-Hydroxysteroid dehydrogenase	3β-HSD	3β-HSD II	*HSD3B2*
17α-Hydroxylase	$P450_{C17}$	CYP17	*CYP17*
21-Hydroxylase	$P450_{C21}$	CYP21A2	*CYP21A2*
11β-Hydroxylase	$P450_{C11}$	CYP11B1	*CYP11B1*
Aldosterone synthase	$P450_{C11AS}$	CYP11B2	*CYP11B2*

Figure 5.
Synthesis of the adrenal cortical hormones.

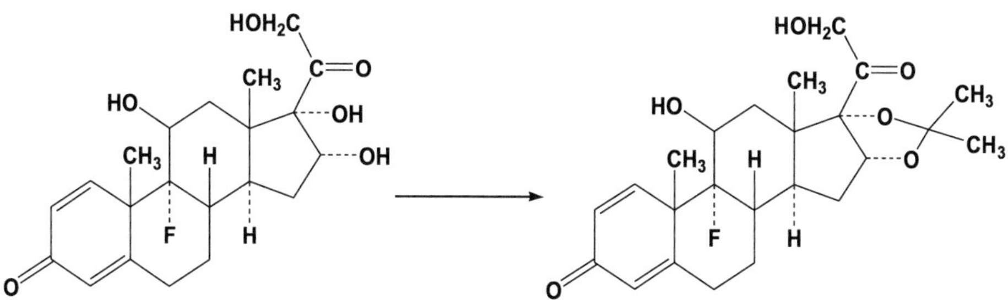

Triamcinolone → Triamcinolone Acetonide

Triamcinolone is converted to acetonide derivative (ketal) by reaction of acetone in the presence of strong acid. The latter is used only locally (topically) [2, 14–16].

They include also 6 α-methyl (methyl prednisolone); 16 α-methyl (Dexamethasone, Alclomethasone, Flumethasone) and 16 β-methyl (Betamethasone, Diflorasone, Paramethasone, Beclomethasone) [2, 3, 14–16, 23].

Other substituents have been found to significantly increase both glucocorticoid and mineralocorticoid activities: 1-ene; 2 α-methyl; 9 α-fluoro; 9 α-chloro; and 21-hydroxy [2, 3, 14–16].

In every case a 16-hydroxy or methyl (to eliminate salt retention) has been combined with another substituent to increase glucocorticoid or anti-inflammatory activity [2, 3, 14–16].

A primary goal of these highly anti-inflammatory drugs has been to increase topical potency [6, 7, 12].

2.5 Risk of systemic absorption

Except for fludrocortisones, the topical corticosteroids do not cause absorption effects when used on small areas of intact skin [6, 7, 12].

The adrenocortical steroids are contraindicated or should be used with great caution in patients having: [2, 3, 6–8, 10–12, 24, 25].

1. Peptic ulcer (in which the steroids may cause hemorrhage)

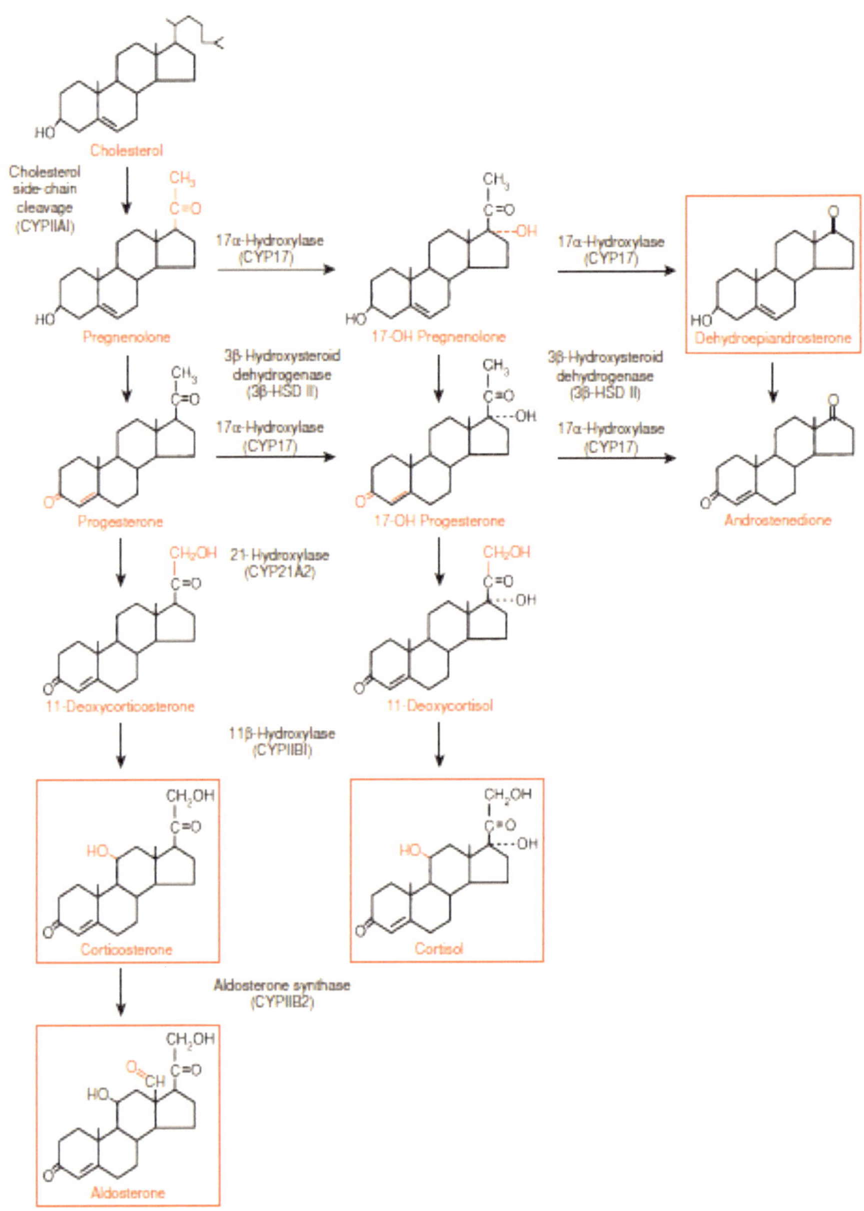

Figure 6.
The synthesis of steroids in the adrenal cortex.

2. Heart disease

3. Infections (the glucocorticoids suppress the body's normal infection-fighting processes)

4. Psychosis (since behavioral disturbances may occur during steroid therapy)

5. Diabetes (the glucocorticoids increase glucose production, so more insulin may be needed)

DOI: http://dx.doi.org/10.5772/intechopen.106785

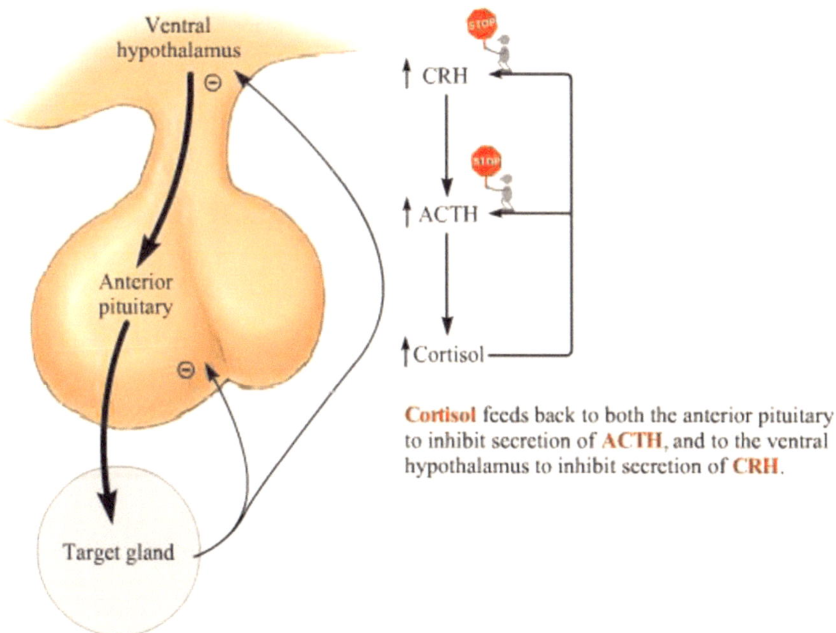

Figure 7.
Cortisol *feeds back to both the anterior pituitary to inhibit secretion of* ***ACTH****, and to the ventral hypothalamus to inhibit secretion of* ***CRH****.*

6. Glaucoma

7. Osteoporosis

8. Herpes simplex involving the cornea

When glucocorticoids are topically administrated, their anti-inflammatory action can mask symptoms of infection.

If absolutely necessary to use the glucocorticoids topically during pregnancy, they should be limited to small areas of intact skin and used for a limited time.

3. The adrenal glands

3.1 Introduction

Pyramid-shaped organs in pairs.

Placed on each kidney's upper poles.

3–5 cm in length on average, weighing 1.5–2.5 gm.

The outer cortex, which is composed primarily of mesodermal tissue and makes about 90% of the weight of the adrenals [26].

The inner medulla (derived from a subpopulation of neural crest).

The adrenal gland is made up of the cortex and medulla. The cortex produces steroid hormones including glucocorticoids, mineralocorticoids, and adrenal

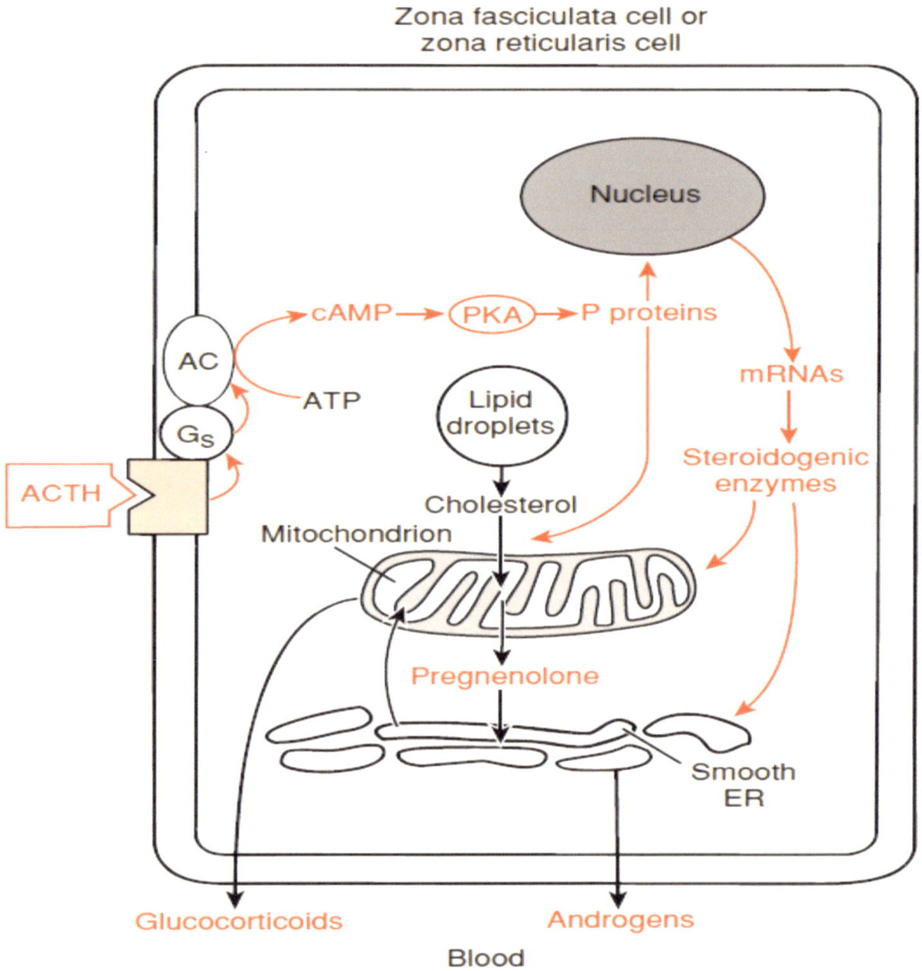

Figure 8.
ACTH's primary effects on steroidogenesis.

androgens, and the medulla produces the catecholamines, epinephrine, and norepinephrine [26].

The body's adaptive response to stress is regulated by the adrenal glands' role in maintaining homeostasis in maintaining the balance of Na and K in the body's water blood pressure regulation [26].

3.2 The main hormones

1. The hormones called steroid (glucocorticoids, mineralocorticoids, androgens).

2. Secondly, catecholamines (norepinephrine, epinephrine).

The two different embryologic origins of the AG have an impact on the mechanisms that each of the two components uses to regulate the production of hormones [17, 26].

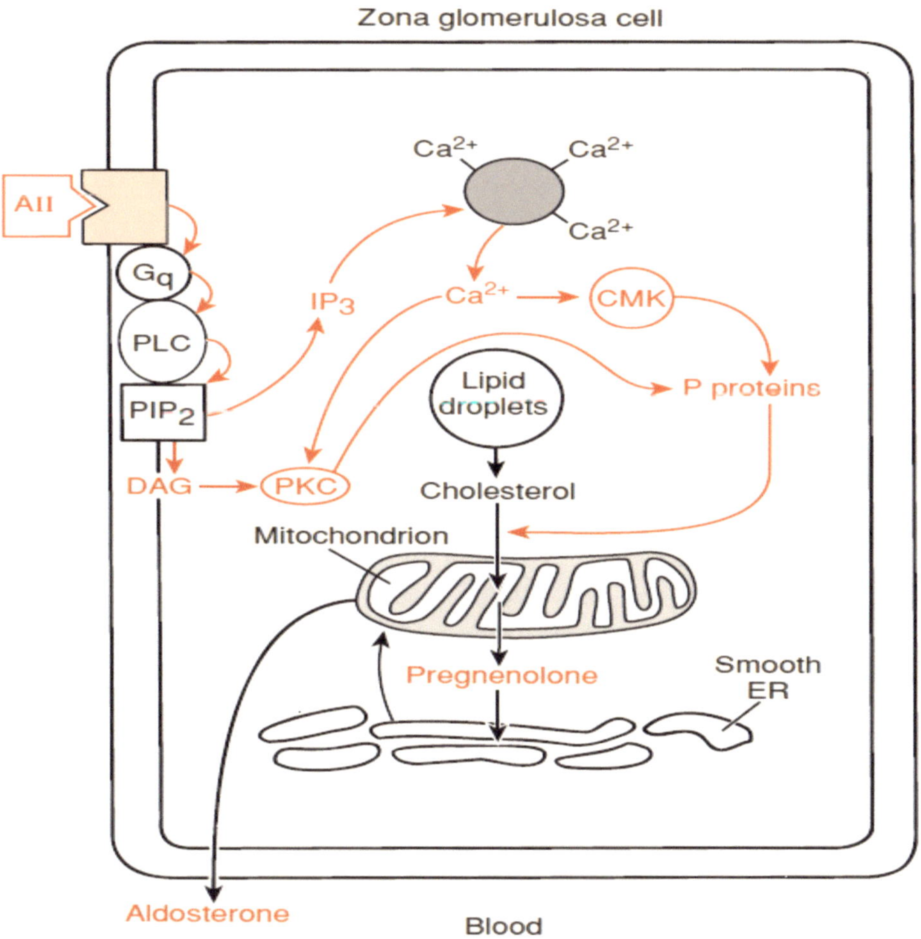

Figure 9.
The impact of angiotensin II on the production of aldosterone.

3.3 Functional anatomy and zonation

Three histologically distinct zones can be found in the adrenal cortex, arranged from outside to inside [27]:

- zona glomerulosa.
- zonafasciculata.
- zonareticularis.

The adrenal cortex secretes the following hormones:

- glucocorticoids.
- aldosterone.

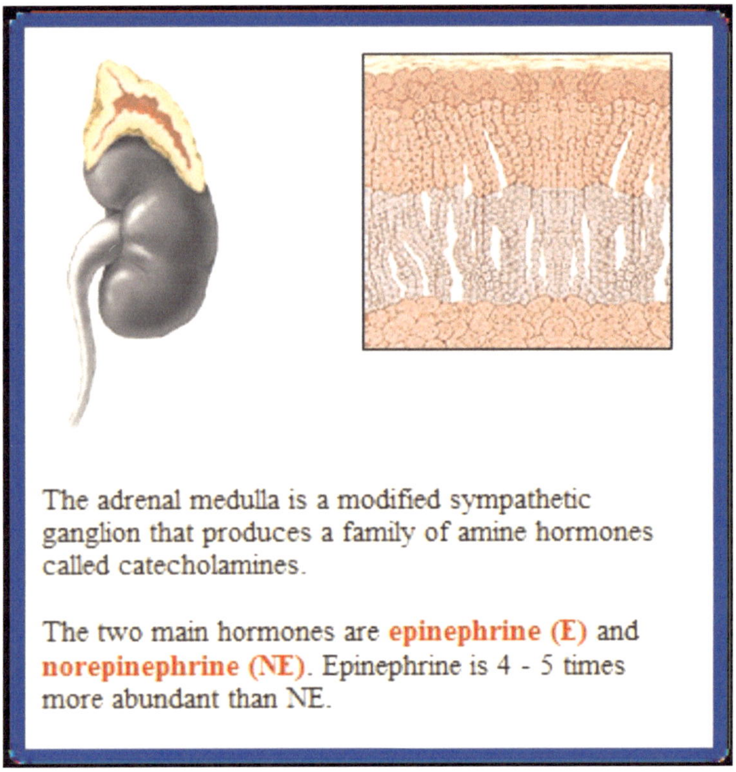

Figure 10.
The adrenal medulla is a modified sympathetic ganglion that produces a family of amine hormones called catecholamines. The two main hormones are epinephrine (E) and norepinephrine (NE). Epinephrine is 4-5 times more abundant than NE. The adrenal medulla [17, 18].

α-Adrenergic mediated	β-Adrenergic mediated
Vasoconstriction	Vasodilation
Iris dilation	Cardioacceleration
Intestinal relaxation	Increased myocardial strength
Intestinal sphincter contraction	Intestinal and bladder wall relaxation
Pilomotor contraction	Uterus relaxation
Bladder sphincter contraction	Bronchodilation
Bronchoconstriction	Calorigenesis
Uterine smooth muscle contraction	Glycogenolysis
Cardiac contractility	Lipolysis
Hepatic glucose production	

Figure 11.
Catecholamine physiologic effects [17, 18].

Liver	Stimulation of glycogenolysis
	Stimulation of gluconeogenesis
Skeletal muscle	Simulation of glycogenolysis
Adipose tissue	Simulation of glycogenolysis
	Stimulation of triglyceride lipolysis
Pancreatic islets	Inhibition of insulin secretion by beta cells
	Stimulation of glucagon secretion by alpha cells

Figure 12.
Catecholamine-mediated responses to hypoglycemia [17, 18].

effect	epinephrine	norepinephrine
peripheral resistance	-	+++
systolic BP	++	+++
diastolic BP	0-	+++
cardiac output	++	-
vasodilation	-	0
glycogenolysis	+++	+
lipolysis	+++	+++
bronchodilation	++	0

Figure 13.
Effects of epinephrine vs. norepinephrine [17, 18]. "–" negative inhibitory effect; "+" positive stimulatory effect; and "0" no effect.

3.4 Zonation

The adrenal cortex's zonafasciculata and zonareticularis are where the glucocorticoids cortisol and corticosterone, as well as the androgen dehydroepiandrosterone, are synthesized [27].

The zonaglomerulosa of the adrenal cortex is where mineralocorticoid aldosterone is made [27].

3.5 Synthesis of the adrenal cortical hormones

Four CYP enzymes (cytochrome P450 enzymes = a large family of oxidative enzymes with a maximum 450 nm absorbance when complexed with carbon monoxide) convert cholesterol into adrenal steroid hormones [28]. Cholesterol esters stored in the cells are used to synthesize the adrenal cortical hormones [28].

LDL particles in the blood are the main source of stored cholesterol, but the AG can also produce it entirely from scratch using acetate [28].

The first step in the synthesis of all adrenal steroids, which happens in each of the three zones of the cortex, is the conversion of cholesterol to pregnenolone in mitochondria. Enzymes that produce steroids [28].

3.6 Genetic defects in adrenal steroidogenesis

Can result in either relative or absolute deficiencies in the enzymes necessary for the biosynthesis of steroid hormones [29].

Changes in the types and quantities of steroid hormones secreted by the adrenal cortex are the direct results of these defects. In the end, disease results [29].

The majority of steroidogenic enzyme-related genetic flaws hinder cortisol production [29].

A decrease in blood cortisol levels prompts the release of ACTH, which has a growth-promoting effect on the adrenal cortex, causing either congenital adrenal hyperplasia or adrenal hypertrophy [29].

3.7 Transport of adrenal steroids in blood

A steroid hormone is prevented from being absorbed by cells or from being excreted in the urine by binding to a circulating protein molecule [18].

The blood is cleared of circulating steroid hormone molecules that are not bound to plasma proteins because they are free to interact with cell receptors [18].

Bound hormone separates from its binding protein and adds more free hormone to the system [18].

The half-lives of adrenal steroid hormones in the body are very long (from many minutes to hours) [18].

3.8 Metabolism of adrenal steroids

After being structurally altered to reduce their hormone activity and increase their water solubility, adrenal steroid hormones are primarily excreted from the body through the urine (primarily in the liver) [29]. Adrenal steroids are primarily metabolized in the liver where they are conjugated to glucuronic acid and eliminated in the urine [29].

3.9 Control over the production of adrenal steroids

By increasing intracellular cAMP, ACTH increases glucocorticoid and androgen synthesis in the zonafasciculata and zonareticularis of the adrenal cortex (cAMPactivates protein kinase A, which phosphorylates proteins that regulate steroidogenesis) [18].

On these cells, ACTH also has a trophic effect [18].

Angiotensin II increases cytosolic calcium and activates protein kinase C in the cells of the zonaglomerulosa to stimulate aldosterone synthesis [18].

ACTH's primary effects on steroidogenesis [18].

When ACTH binds to plasma membrane receptors, stimulatory G proteins connect those receptors to adenylyl cyclase (AC) (Gs).

Protein kinase A (PKA) is activated by cAMP in the cells, which phosphorylates specific proteins (PProteins). The expression of the genes for steroidogenic enzymes is stimulated and steroidogenesis is presumably started by these proteins.

The expression of the genes for steroidogenic enzymes is stimulated and steroidogenesis is presumably started by these proteins [18].

The impact of angiotensin II on the production of aldosterone [18].

Angiotensin II (AII) binds to receptors on the plasma membrane of zonaglomerulosa cells. Phospholipase C (PLC), which is connected to the angiotensin II receptor by G proteins, is activated as a result (Gq) [18].

In the plasma, PLC hydrolyzes phosphatidylinositol 4,5 bisphosphate (PIP2) membrane, resulting in the production of IP3 and diacylglycerol (DAG) [18].

3.10 Intracellularly bound Ca2 is moved by IP3

Protein kinase C (PKC) and calmodulin-dependent protein kinase are both activated by an increase in Ca2 and DAG (CMK) [18]. These enzymes phosphorylate the proteins (P-Proteins) that start the synthesis of aldosterone [18].

4. Process of action

Target cells' cytosol contains glucocorticoid receptors, which glucocorticoids bind to [18]. The glucocorticoid-bound receptor moves to the nucleus where it attaches to DNA glucocorticoid response elements to alter the transcription of particular genes [18]. The body must have access to glucocorticoids in order to adjust to stress, injury, and fasting [18].

Glucocorticoids

Very powerful and responsible for about 95% of all glucocorticoid activity is cortisol [18].

About 4% of the total glucocorticoid activity is provided by corticosterone, which is significantly less potent than cortisol [18].

Cortisone, which is nearly as potent as cortisol [18].

Synthetic, four times as potent as cortisol, prednisone [18].

Synthetic methylprednisone, which has five times the potency of cortisol [18] (Synthetic, 30 times more potent than cortisol) Dexamethasone [18].

Glucocorticoids' effects [18].

Catabolic, anti-anabolic, and diabetogenic effects on metabolism.

Glucocorticoids' Anti-Inflammatory Properties.

The Immune System's Impact.

Protection of the Norepinephrine-Induced Vascular Response.

Stress Glucocorticoids.

Glucocorticoid Secretion Control.

Glucocorticoids Are Involved in the Responses to Injury, Stress, and Fasting [18].

Effects of cortisol on the metabolism of carbohydrates: [18]

Stimulation of Gluconeogenesis - Cortisol increases the enzymes needed in the liver cells to convert amino acids into glucose [18].

Cortisol causes the extrahepatic tissues, primarily muscle, to release amino acids [18].

Cells' Utilization of Glucose is Reduced [18].

"Adrenal Diabetes" and Increased Blood Glucose Concentration [18].

Cortisol's Impact on Protein Metabolism [18].

Protein Cellular Reductionin.

Plasma and Liver Protein Levels are Raised by Cortisol a rise in blood amino acids, a decline in amino acid transport into extrahepatic cells, and an improvement in transport into hepatic cells.

Cortisol's Impact on Fat Metabolism [18].

Mobilization of Fatty Acids Excess Cortisol Leads to Obesity.

Cortisol Helps the Body Fight Stress and Inflammation.

Effects of High Cortisol Levels on Inflammation.

Cortisol Prevents the Development of Inflammation through Other Effects and Lysosome Stabilization.

Cortisol Leads to Inflammation Healing.

The Inflammatory Response to Allergic Reactions is Blocked by Cortisol.

Effects of cortisol in reducing inflammation.

The lysosomal membranes are stabilized by cortisol.

Capillary permeability is lessened by cortisol.

White blood cell migration into the inflamed area and phagocytosis of the aged cells are both decreased by cortisol.

Cortisol significantly reduces lymphocyte production by suppressing the immune system.

Cortisol reduces interleukin-1 release from white blood cells, which is the primary mechanism by which it lowers fever.

Mineralocorticoids [18].

Aldosterone (very potent, accounts for about 90 percent of all mineralocorticoid activity).

Deoxycorticosterone (1/30 as powerful as aldosterone, but secreted in very small amounts).

Corticosterone (slight mineralocorticoid activity).

9α-Fluorocortisol (synthetic, slightly more potent than aldosterone).

Cortisol (very slight mineralocorticoid activity, but large quantity secreted).

Cortisone (slight mineralocorticoid activity).

Mineralocorticoids' effects [18].

Aldosterone stimulates sodium reabsorption in the kidneys by the distal tubule and collecting duct of the nephron and promotes the excretion of potassium and hydrogen ions, according to its physiological action.

Since potassium directly affects zona glomerulosa cells, an increase in the concentration of potassium in extracellular fluid stimulates aldosterone secretion.

Aldosterone Secretion Control.

The extracellular fluid's increased potassium ion concentration significantly boosts aldosterone secretion.

Aldosterone secretion is also significantly increased by an increase in the extracellular fluid's angiotensin II concentration.

Aldosterone secretion is very slightly reduced when the extracellular fluid's sodium ion concentration rises.

Aldosterone secretion requires ACTH from the anterior pituitary gland, but it has little impact on regulating the rate of secretion in most.

The catecholamines epinephrine (adrenaline) and norepinephrine (noradrenaline).

Four adrenergic receptors (alpha 1, 2, beta 1, 2) interact with catecholamines to mediate the effects of the hormones on cells.

Catecholamines have immediate and extensive effects.

Catecholamines are released from the chromaffin cells as a result of impulses generated in the cholinergic preganglionic fibers that innervate them by stimuli like injury, rage, pain, cold, strenuous exercise, and hypoglycemia.

Catecholamines promote the production of glucose in the liver, the release of lactate from muscle, and the breakdown of fat in adipose tissue to combat hypoglycemia.

5. Conclusion

The body's defense mechanisms depend heavily on the adrenal glands.

They trigger physiological adjustments that are required to combat changes in the environment outside the body. They also secrete a number of vital hormones that are crucial for maintaining a healthy immune system, metabolic rate, and salt and water balance in the body. Additionally protecting the body from stress. High levels of glucocorticosteroid production in response to stress can result in a 95 percent reduction in thymus gland size. It has not yet been completely determined how glucocorticoid stimulation protects against stress.

Author details

Ali Gamal Ahmed Al-kaf
Faculty of Pharmacy, Medicinal Chemistry Department, Sana'a University, Yemen

*Address all correspondence to: alialkaf21@gmail.com

References

[1] Nigam LK, Vanikar AV, Patel RD, Kanodia KV, Suthar KS. Pathology Associated with Hormones of Adrenal Cortex. Submitted: September 8th, 2018; Reviewed: January 29th, 2019; Published: November 27th, 2019. DOI: 10.5772/intechopen.84815

[2] Wilson, Gisvold's. Textbook of Organic Medicinal and Pharmaceutical Chemistry. 12th ed. New York: Lippincott; 2011. p. 1022

[3] Belikov VG. Pharmaceutical chemistry. Pyatigorsk: Pyatigorsk press; 2003;**3**:720

[4] Wagner G, Khumstedt H. Pharmaceutische Chemie. Berlin; 1978

[5] Russian Pharmacopoeia. Vol. 12. Moscow: Moscow Press; 2008. p. 704

[6] Martindale: The Extra pharmacopoeia. Edited by Sweetman SC. 36th ed. Vol. 20. pages 3709. London: Pharmaceutical Press; 2009

[7] Mashkovskiy MD. The Medicinal Remedies. Moscow: OOO "Publishers New Wave"; 2005. p. 1200

[8] Goodman, Gilman's. The Pharmacological Basis of Therapeutics. 11 ed. USA; 2006. p. 2021

[9] Wells BG, Dipiro JT, Schwinghammer TL, Dipiro CV. Pharmacotherapy Handbook. 7 ed. USA; 2009. p. 1066

[10] Goldman's Cecil Medicine. 24th ed. 2012

[11] Roche VF. The chemically elegant proton pump inhibitors. American Journal of Pharmaceutical Education. 2006;**70**(5):101. Available from: http://www.ncbi.nlm.nih.gov/pmc/articles/PMC1637016/figure/F6/

[12] Bennett PN, Brown MJ. Clinical Pharmacology. 9 ed. Spain: Churchill Livingstone; 2003. p. 789

[13] Davidson's Principles and Practice of Medicine. 20th ed. Vol. 8882011

[14] Nadendla RR. Priciples of Organic Medicinal Chemistry. New Delhi: New Age Publishers; 2005. p. 322

[15] Kar A. Medicinal Chemistry. 4 ed. Vol. 933. India; 2007

[16] Williams DA, Lemke TL. Foye's Principles of Medicinal Chemistry. 6th ed. USA; 2008

[17] Paravati S, Rosani A, Warrington SJ. StatPearls. Treasure Island (FL): StatPearls Publishing; 2021. Physiology, Catecholamines. [PubMed]

[18] Nussey S, Whitehead S. Endocrinology. An Integrated Approach. Oxford: BIOS Scientific Publishers; 2001. ISBN-10: 1-85996-252-1

[19] Thomas G. Medicinal Chemistry. 2nd ed. England: John Wiley & Sons Ltd; 2007. p. 648

[20] Donald JA. Burger's Medicinal Chemistry and Drug Discovery. 6 ed. Vol. 1-6. USA; 2003

[21] Voge L, Gerhard H. Drug Discovery and Evalution. 2 ed. Germany; 2002. p. 1408

[22] Patrick GL. An Introduction to Medicinal Chemistry. 2 ed. Vol. 621. India; 2003

[23] Negwer M. Organic –Chemical Drugs and Their Synonyms. Band 1-111. Berlin; 1987

[24] Drug Information for the Health Care Professional. 22nd ed. Vol. 1. New York; 2002. p. 3291

[25] Kumar, Clark's. Clinical Medicine. 8th ed. 2012

[26] Megha R, Wehrle CJ, Kashyap S, Leslie SW. StatPearls. Treasure Island (FL): StatPearls Publishing; 2021. Anatomy, Abdomen and Pelvis, Adrenal Glands (Suprarenal Glands) [PubMed]

[27] Xing Y, Lerario AM, Rainey W, Hammer GD. Development of adrenal cortex zonation. Endocrinology and Metabolism Clinics of North America. 2015;**44**(2):243-274. [PMC free article] [PubMed]

[28] Ortsäter H, Sjöholm Å, Rafacho A. Regulation of Glucocorticoid Receptor Signaling and the Diabetogenic Effects of Glucocorticoid Excess. Submitted: July 11th2012. Reviewed: July 21st, 2012 Published: October 3rd, 2012. DOI: 10.5772/51759

[29] Turcu AF, Auchus RJ. Adrenal steroidogenesis and congenital adrenal hyperplasia. Endocrinology and Metabolism Clinics in North America. 2015;**44**(2):275-296. DOI: 10.1016/j.ecl.2015.02.002

Section 2

Adrenal Gland Pathology

Chapter 3

Combination of High Prevalence Sign/Symptom Pairs: An Approach to the Diagnosis of Cushing's Syndrome

Aída Verónica Araya, Claudio Liberman, Claudia Munizaga, Pedro Pineda, Marcela Barberán, Francisco Cordero, Alejandra Lanas and Luís Toro

Abstract

Most of the clinical features of Cushing's syndrome (CS) are nonspecific and could be present in obesity, particularly when this condition is associated with metabolic syndrome. Our objective was to evaluate the frequency of clinical manifestations and changes in general laboratory tests, in patients with confirmed endogenous CS, to identify diagnostic dyads. We evaluated in each patient the rate of coexistence of 2 elements either: symptoms, clinical signs, or laboratory alteration. The prevalence of a combined pair of clinical features or dyad in over 30% of the cases, was considered clinically significant. Fourteen dyads were identified as clinically relevant. Facies + buffalo hump; facies + eosinopenia; buffalo hump + supraclavicular fat pads and facies + supraclavicular fat pads, were present in over 50% of cases. Facies + muscular atrophy; centripetal fat distribution + muscular atrophy and facies + striae were present in 42–49%. Hirsutism/acne + eosinopenia; buffalo hump + eosinopenia; muscular atrophy+ eosinopenia; eosinopenia + accelerated weight gain; buffalo hump + muscular atrophy; hirsutism/acne + muscular atrophy and hirsutism/acne + supraclavicular fat pads, were observed in 33–38% of patients. Its application will facilitate the correct diagnosis of CS.

Keywords: Cushing, Cushing's syndrome, Cushing's syndrome/diagnosis, dyads, eosinopenia, muscle weakness, muscle atrophy

1. Introduction

Classical manifestations of Cushing's syndrome (CS) are related to cortisol excess. Frequent physical signs are moon face and plethora, buffalo hump, supraclavicular fat pads, central obesity, width and dark red striae, thin limbs, thin skin, hirsutism, and acne. Frequent symptoms are accelerated weight gain, muscular weakness, amenorrhea, pathological fractures/osteoporosis. In general laboratory tests, alterations secondary to hypercortisolism can be found (examples: hyperglycemia, hypertriglyceridemia, hypokalemia, low eosinophils, and lymphocytes count.

Nevertheless, most of the clinical features of CS are nonspecific and could be found in obesity, particularly, in association with metabolic syndrome. For this reason, diagnosis is often overlooked, and treatment is delayed unless the evaluation is done by an expert endocrinologist.

A meta-analysis published in 2020 (which included 44 studies) showed that mean time delay to diagnosis CS was 34 months. This was shorter in ectopic CS (14 months) compared with adrenal CS (30 months) and pituitary Cushing's (38 months), probably due to the more aggressive behavior of these neoplasms [1].

For this reason, it seems necessary to establish clinical features of suspicion of this disorder that can be used by non-specialists.

More than fifty years ago, it was reported that in about 50% of patients with suspected CS, the diagnosis could be confirmed or excluded using clinical or general laboratory tests with greater accuracy than steroid screening [2].

Nevertheless, with the increasing prevalence of obesity and its associated metabolic disorders, experts questioned the use of the classical clinical parameters and validated only specific signs related to hypercortisolism (osteopenia, thin skin, and proximal muscular weakness). When they are used to confirm or discard CS diagnosis, the probability is 95% [3, 4].

Over decades, different authors have proposed methods to approach clinical diagnosis of this syndrome (**Table 1**). In the sixties, Nugent et al. studied the incidence of

Reference	n° patients	Discriminatory signs/ symptoms	Parameter	Estimated value for diagnosis of CS
Nugent, 1964 [2]	38 CS/73 Non-CS	Weakness, ecchymoses, edema, low serum potassium	Probability	0.9 to ≥ 0.99
Ross, 1982 [4]	70 CS/159 Non-CS	Bruising, myopathy, hypertension, plethora, edema, hirsutism, red striae	Discriminant index*	>2
Schneider, 2013 [5]	73 CS/369 Non-CS	Recurrent infections, red striae, amenorrhea, abdominal fat distribution, plethora, muscular weakness, hirsutism	Discriminant index**	≥ 2
León-Justel, 2016 [6]	389 at risk of CS	Muscular atrophy, osteoporosis, dorsocervical fat pad	ROC analysis score	4
Loriaux, 2017 [3]	Estimated prevalence 0.2%	Thin skin, osteopenia, ecchymoses	Probability***	95%

**Index calculated by dividing the prevalence of each feature in CS by its prevalence in reference [2] of 159 mostly obese patients in whom the diagnosis of Cushing's syndrome was suspected but not biochemically substantiated.*
***Index calculated by dividing the prevalence in authors series with the prevalence reported in reference [4].*
****Obtained using a probability of 0.2% and a likelihood ratio of 116 for thin skin, 18 for osteopenia, and 4 for ecchymoses*

Table 1.
Diagnostic models of Cushing syndrome based on prevalent signs and symptoms.

different signs in patients with and without the syndrome. They reported that the more significant findings were osteoporosis, central or generalize obesity, weakness, plethora, leukocytosis (≥11,000/μL), acne, striae (red or purple), diastolic hypertension (≥105 mmHg), edema, hirsutism, ecchymoses, and low serum potassium (≤3.6 mEq/L). These signs were used to calculate the probability of CS. The results suggested that diagnosis could be confirmed or excluded with a high degree of confidence in at least half of patients with suspected CS [2].

In the early 80s, another paper showed that bruising, muscle weakness, and hypertension were the most discriminating features of CS (discriminant index over 4) [5].

Other authors evaluated the prevalence of signs and symptoms in a series of 73 cases of CS and calculated a discriminant index. The signs and symptoms, with a higher index (2 or greater) were recurrent infections, red striae, amenorrhea, abdominal fat distribution, plethora, muscular weakness, and hirsutism [6].

Another group developed a risk score to predict CS in a population of over 300 subjects at-risk. They propose two models, one based on the assessment of clinical symptoms and signs, and in the other, late-night salivary cortisol (LNSC) determination was added to the clinical features. The multivariate logistic regression analysis showed that muscular atrophy, osteoporosis, and dorsal cervical fat pad remained independent variables associated with CS. The ROC analysis showed that a score of 4 resulted in sensitivity and specificity of 96.2% and 82.9%, respectively. With this cut-off value, 83% of subjects without CS were correctly identified and only one of 26 CS was missed. However, they reported several false positives, mainly related with the LNSC level [7].

Applying technology, in a study of 20 patients with CS, a facial appearance classification software was tested to discriminate patients with Cushing from healthy controls. The software correctly classified 85% of patients and 95% of controls, with a total classification accuracy of 91.7%. Nevertheless, this study only evaluated women, which limited its utility [8].

On the other hand, within general laboratory tests, impaired blood glucose and abnormal lipid levels may be present in a high percentage of the obese population, however, low potassium levels in absence of diuretic use and low eosinophil count may be typical manifestations of hypercortisolism.

Eosinopenia is defined as a reduction of circulating eosinophils < 10/μL or < 0.1% of total leukocyte count. In physiological conditions, during acute stress, eosinopenia is mediated by adrenal glucocorticoids and epinephrine. In patients treated with corticosteroids, eosinopenia would result from an impairment in the release of these cells from the bone marrow and its sequestration of the blood pool [9]. Chronic hypercortisolemia in CS can explain this typical finding which should be taken into account when evaluating a suspected case.

Because laboratory tests performed to confirm the diagnosis of CS are not routinary done and are not widely available, the selection of cases that requires evaluation should be done by a specialist but given a large number of obese patients, this is impracticable. For this reason, combinations of signs, symptoms, and general laboratory tests could be a useful tool for clinicians when CS is suspected.

Our objective was to evaluate the frequency of clinical signs, symptoms, and biochemical alterations in patients treated in a single center with a confirmed endogenous CS and identify dyads of specific symptoms and/or signs.

2. Methodology

This was a retrospective review of clinical records, laboratory tests, radiological exams, and biopsies from patients treated in one university center in the period 1980–2017. We excluded patients under corticosteroid therapy, those whose physical examination was not performed by an endocrinologist and with incomplete records. At least two of the following tests confirmed the diagnosis of CS: free urinary cortisol (FUC), overnight 1 mg Dexamethasone suppression test (Nugent's test), and LNSC. The etiology of CS was confirmed by the following: plasma ACTH, hormonal functional tests, and radiological exams. Operated patients had a confirmatory biopsy. This protocol was approved by the local scientific Ethics Committee.

We determined patient characteristics, including age, gender, reason for consultation, features at physical examination, and general laboratory tests, establishing the frequency for each parameter.

We evaluated the rate of coexistence of two features either: symptoms, clinical signs, or laboratory alterations in each patient. A prevalence of a combined pair or dyad in over 30% of the cases was considered clinically relevant. Finally, according to expert endocrinologist opinion and based on scientific literature on the subject, we selected diagnostic dyads with the more specific features of hypercortisolism. Statistical analysis was performed using STATA SE v 15.0 software (StataCorp LLC).

2.1 Definitions of some specific signs of hypercortisolism

- Accelerated weight gain: weight increase over 7–10% in less than 3 months.
- Changes in fat distribution: Increase of thoracoabdominal fat (centripetal fat depot) and decrease in buttocks and limbs.
- Buffalo hump: fat accumulation in dorsocervical region.
- Supraclavicular fat pads: fat accumulation in supraclavicular hollows.
- Striae: dark red or violet, ≥ 1 cm width, mainly in abdomen (paraumbilical and flanks), inner thighs, and arms.
- Thin skin/Ecchymoses: translucent appearance, frail / 3 or more ecchymoses.
- Muscular atrophy: decrease in quadriceps, buttocks, and biceps muscle mass on palpation.
- Hirsutism: characteristics and distribution of body hair according to Ferriman Gallwey score [10].
- Eosinopenia: eosinophils count $< 10/\mu L$ or $< 0.1\%$ of total leukocyte count.

3. Results

In the analyzed period, 102 patients, 89 women (87.2%), 36.9 ± 13 years old (15–72 yo), had confirmed CS.

The etiology of CS was pituitary (68%), adrenal (23%), and ectopic ACTH (9%).

Clinical characteristics are shown in **Table 2**. The more frequent clinical symptoms were accelerated weight increase (57.3%), hirsutism and/or acne (23%), and muscular weakness (22%). At physical examination, the most frequent signs were moon face (90%), centripetal fat depot (78.4%), buffalo hump (65.7%), supraclavicular fat pads (53.9%), hirsutism and/or acne (mainly in women) (65%), systolic and/or diastolic hypertension (60%), muscular atrophy (52%) and striae (42%). At the laboratory tests, we found eosinophils count < 0.1% of total leukocytes in 84.2%.

From 520 combinations of data pairs, we obtained 18 dyads present in over 30% of cases (**Table 3**). From these, we selected 14 dyads which feature combinations were considered more specific to hypercortisolism. Facies + buffalo hump; facies + eosinopenia; buffalo hump + supraclavicular fat pads and facies + supraclavicular fat pads, were present in over 50% of cases. Facies + muscular atrophy; centripetal fat distribution + muscular atrophy and facies + striae were present in 42–49%. Hirsutism/acne + eosinopenia; buffalo hump + eosinopenia; muscular atrophy+ eosinopenia; eosinopenia + accelerated weight gain; buffalo hump + muscular atrophy; hirsutism/acne + muscular atrophy and hirsutism/acne + supraclavicular fat pads, were observed in 33–38% of patients.

4. Discussion

Cushing's Syndrome represents a clinical challenge even for specialists. As we mentioned before, many features related to hypercortisolism could be found in other clinical conditions. Some of them correspond to pseudo-Cushing's states. This condition shares clinical signs of CS and equivocal evidence of hypercortisolism in laboratory tests [11]. One study disclosed that obesity (BMI>30 kg/m^2) was significantly more frequent in pseudo-Cushing than in CS and only ecchymoses and osteoporosis were more frequent in CS [12]. Another study showed that obesity, moon face, and buffalo hump were present in over 50% of pseudo-Cushing's patients [13].

Nonetheless, even in this condition, a meticulous clinical evaluation could improve diagnostic accuracy and the finding of combination of frequent signs, symptoms, and biochemical tests could be the best approach to continue with more specific evaluations.

Interestingly, classical signs of hypercortisolism were present in a high proportion of our cases, as is shown in **Table 2**. Accelerated weight gain and change in body fat distribution were frequent causes of consultation and feature at physical examination (58% and 78% respectively).

In vitro and *in vivo* studies have shown that glucocorticoids (GCs) increase hypothalamic endocannabinoids. GCs and cannabinoids have been shown to increase hypothalamic adenine monophosphate protein kinase-A (AMPK) activity, resulting in increased appetite. Moreover, GCs have been shown to upregulate gene expression of orexigenic peptides such as Y neuropeptide (NPY) and agouti-related peptides. This could explain cravings for fat and carbohydrates observed in endogenous GCs excess states as Cushing's disease [14].

Some studies in human healthy controls or subjects with inflammatory conditions evaluated the effect of short-term use of oral GCs on energy intake, body weight, body composition, or appetite but, results have not been conclusive [15].

Still, more studies are necessary to establish the effects of long-term use of oral GCs and endogenous hypercortisolism, on appetite and dietary intake.

N	102 (%)
Age (yr)	36.9 ± 13.0
Gender: Females Males	89 (87.3%) 13 (12.7%)
Reason for consultation	
Accelerated weight gain/changes in fat distribution	59 (57.3%)
Muscular weakness	23 (22.1%)
Menstrual disorders	10 (9.7%)
Hirsutism/acne	24 (23.3%)
Hypertension	10 (9.7%)
Hyperglycemia/diabetes/dislipidemia	8 (7.8%)
Osteoporosis/fractures	5 (4.9%)
Skin alterations	8 (7.8%)
Edema	7 (6.8%)
Neuropsyquiatric	5 (4.9%)
Other	12 (11.7%)
Physical examination	
Moon Face	91 (89.2%)
Hirsutism/acne	60 (58.8%)
Buffalo hump	67 (65.7%)
Supraclavicular fat pads	55 (53.9%)
Acanthosis	32 (31.4%)
Centripetal fat distribution	80 (78.4%)
Muscular atrophy	53 (52.0%)
Thin skin/ecchymoses	30 (29.4%)
Striae	43 (42.2%)
Hyperpigmentation	13 (12.7%)
Systolic blood pressure > 140 mm/Hg	62 (62.0%)
Diastolic blood pressure > 90 mm/Hg	57 (57%)
BMI (kg/m^2)	
26–29	26 (26.8%)
30–35	27 (27.8%)
> 35	17 (17.5%)
General Laboratory	
Eosinophil count <10/μL or <0.1% of total leukocyte count	64 (84.2%)
Lymphocytes < 1000/μL	12 (18.5%)
Hyperglycemia	43 (50.0%)

N	**102 (%)**
Hypertriglyceridemia	22 (55.5%)
Hypokalemia	28 (31.1%)

Table 2.
Clinical features in patients with Cushing's syndrome.

Facies + buffalo hump	60.7%
Facies + eosinopenia	54.9%
Buffalo hump + supraclavicular fat pads	52.9%
Facies + supraclavicular fat pads	50.9%
Facies + muscular atrophy	49.0%
Centripetal fat distribution+ muscular atrophy	43.1%
Facies + striae	42.1%
Hirsutism/acne + buffalo hump	38.2%
Hirsutism/acne + eosinopenia	38.2%
Buffalo hump + eosinopenia	36.2%
Systolic hypertension + eosinopenia	35.2%
Muscular atrophy+ eosinopenia	34.3%
Eosinopenia + accelerated weight gain	34.3%
Buffalo hump + muscular atrophy	33.3%
Diastolic hypertension + eosinopenia	33.3%
Muscular atrophy + systolic hypertension	32.3%
Hirsutism/acne + muscular atrophy	31.3%
Hirsutism/acne + supraclavicular fat pads	30.3%

Table 3.
Diagnostic dyads.

On the other hand, changes in fat redistribution are determined by chronic hypercortisolism, leading to an increase in centripetal adiposity and visceral abdominal fat. Regulation of adipose tissue mass is complex and involved mechanisms are multiple and still not completely understood. In general, the effects of GCs on adipose tissue depend on the duration of the exposure to GCs and on the type of adipose tissue considered (subcutaneous or visceral) [16]. Visceral fat would be differentially responsive to GCs than subcutaneous fat. In experimental models, GCs induce the differentiation of preadipocytes, specific to visceral fat, but not for subcutaneous fat. Glucocorticoid receptor expression is higher in visceral than in peripheral subcutaneous fat. Chronic corticoid exposure increases lipogenesis in visceral adipose compartment and increases lipolysis in subcutaneous adipose tissue [17]. Also, there is a higher cortisol production in visceral adipose tissue, due to an increased expression of GC receptors and 11B-hydroxysteroid dehydrogenase type 1 (11BHSD1) enzymatic activity. The 11BHSD1 is widely expressed throughout the body, including liver, visceral and subcutaneous fat, and promotes the conversion of inactive cortisone to cortisol. These mechanisms among others, explain the characteristic phenotype of CS [18].

Another relevant clinical feature is muscle involvement. In our case series, muscle atrophy was present in 52% of cases. In previous reports, the prevalence of muscle weakness or atrophy was 20–45% [6, 7, 12]. Chronic hypercortisolism generally has a more prominent effect on the proximal muscles. GC-induced muscle atrophy affects mainly fast-twitch or type II fibers with less or no impact on type I or slow-twitch fibers. This explains the characteristic findings at physical examination of thin limbs with loss of muscle mass.

GCs reduce skeletal muscle mass both by inhibiting protein synthesis and by increasing the rate of protein degradation. GCs stimulate myostatin, an inhibitory growth factor that downregulates protein synthesis and also, proliferation and differentiation of muscle satellite cells, precursors of skeletal muscle cells. GCs inhibit the transport of amino acids into the muscle and interfere with the stimulatory action of insulin and Insulin-like Growth Factor 1 (IGF1) on the protein synthesis pathways. Moreover, GCs inhibit the production of IGF1 in muscle, which contributes to muscle proteolysis and apoptosis [18]. On the other side, GCs can indirectly affect skeletal muscle by downregulating gonadal function and reducing the expression of the androgen receptor. This would explain the authors' finding of high frequency of myopathy in males compared with females (65% *vs* 45%) [19].

Recently, some researchers compared muscle mass and muscle function in patients with CS and matched obese controls. The CS group showed a significant decrease in muscle function tests (chair rising time and hand grip strength) versus the obese non-CS group. Interestingly, both groups did not show differences in muscle mass, fat mass and waist-to-hip ratio, suggesting that CS could be associated with impaired muscle quality and functional alterations more than in trophic effects [20]. Functional tests could be other clinical tool to objectify the diagnosis of CS.

It is interesting that skin manifestations were not observed with high frequency in our cases (only 29%), as has been reported previously [21]. In that report, they used a caliper to measure the skinfold over the proximal phalanx of the middle finger of the nondominant hand. Our diagnosis was based on observation only. Also, we must consider that our patients have different ethnic backgrounds.

Another issue observed in CS patients is metabolic complications, as hyperglycemia, dyslipidemia and higher cardiovascular risk. These are due to several GCs related actions on the liver, skeletal muscle, pancreas, and adipose tissue [see Ref. 22]. In omental, but not in subcutaneous adipocytes, GCs induce insulin resistance by increasing free fatty acid, inducing deregulation in adipokines secretion, and increasing leptin and resistin levels. IL6 and TNFα receptor 1 are also increased in CS patients compared to BMI-matched controls. In some series, a prevalence of diabetes between 15–45% was reported [6, 7, 12, 19] and 46% of dyslipidemia [7]. In our series, 50% had hyperglycemia and hypertriglyceridemia. It should be mentioned that not all cases had a glucose tolerance test, so this probably underestimated the frequency of hyperglycemic disorders.

A remarkable finding observed, is a decrease in eosinophil count. Eosinopenia/aneosinophilia determined by excess of GCs. has been described for more than 6 decades. Patients with CS may present leukocytosis and neutrophilia and a low lymphocyte and eosinophil count or eosinopenia [9, 23, 24]. In the absence of exogenous corticosteroid use, eosinopenia would be the most specific laboratory finding. Patients with pseudo-Cushing, present various clinical signs and even altered laboratory tests such as FUC or Nugent's test, but do not have eosinopenia [11]. We found an eosinophil count < 0.1% of total leukocyte count in over 80% of cases, unlike lymphopenia, observed only in 18% of patients. Then, we consider eosinopenia a significant diagnostic element.

The association of eosinopenia with signs such as hypertension or hirsutism, which are observed commonly in other pathologies with similar characteristics to CS, like polycystic ovary syndrome (PCOS), leads toward the diagnosis of Cushing's. The combination of hirsutism/acne + eosinopenia and systolic hypertension + eosinopenia were prevalent in CS (38% and 35%).

Decreased bone mass density was frequent in other series [7, 12]. But, in our patients we found osteoporosis only in 5%. However, it should be noted that this was due to the fact that bone densitometry was performed in a minority of cases. Then, this sign was underestimated in our cases and always should be considered if it is present together with any of the diagnostic dyads.

5. Conclusion

We present a casuistry with a large number of patients with a confirmed Cushing's syndrome which makes our findings very significant. The combinations of high-risk clinical pairs or dyads associated with determined disease have been used for the identification of patients at risk of other pathology such as acromegaly [25].

The presence of dyad combinations of clinical features may be a useful tool in a practical clinical setting, to assist physicians in identifying patients at risk of CS, without requiring complex or expensive tests.

With training, that allows recognizing the specific signs of hypercortisolism and general laboratory tests, the use of these sign/symptom dyads (shown in **Table 3**), will facilitate that the correct diagnosis of CS can be reached with high certainty.

An early diagnosis and treatment of Cushing syndrome, most probably will reduce the severe comorbidities associated with this condition and will improve the prognosis of these patients.

Acknowledgements

To the neurosurgery team of the University of Chile Clinical Hospital, who referred many patients for evaluation.

Conflict of interest

The authors declare no conflict of interest.

Author details

Aída Verónica Araya[1,2]*, Claudio Liberman[1], Claudia Munizaga[2], Pedro Pineda[1], Marcela Barberán[2], Francisco Cordero[1], Alejandra Lanas[1] and Luís Toro[3]

1 Endocrinology Section, University of Chile Clinical Hospital, Chile

2 Endocrinology Unit, Las Condes Clinic, Santiago, Chile

3 Center for Advanced Clinical Research, University of Chile Clinical Hospital, Chile

*Address all correspondence to: draveronicaaraya@gmail.com

References

[1] Rubinstein G, Osswald A, Hoster E, Losa M, Elenkova A, Zacharieva S, et al. Time to diagnosis in Cushing's Syndrome: A meta-analysis based on 5367 patients. The Journal of Clinical Endocrinology and Metabolism. 2020; **105**:1-11

[2] Nugent CA, Warner HR, Dunn JT, Tyler FH. Probability theory in the diagnosis of Cushing's Syndrome. The Journal of Clinical Endocrinology and Metabolism. 1964;**24**:621-627. DOI: 10.1210/jcem-24-7-621

[3] Loriaux DL. Diagnosis and Differential Diagnosis of Cushing's Syndrome. The New England Journal of Medicine. 2017;**376**:1451-1459. DOI: 10.1056/NEJMra1505550

[4] Baid SK, Rubino D, Sinaii N, Ramsey S, Frank A, Nieman LK. Specificity of screening tests for Cushing's syndrome in an overweight and obese population. The Journal of Clinical Endocrinology and Metabolism. 2009;**94**:3857-1864. DOI: 10.1210/jc.2008-2766

[5] Ross EJ, Linch DC. Cushing's syndrome—Killing disease: Discriminatory value of signs and symptoms aiding early diagnosis. Lancet. 1982;**8299**:646-649. DOI: 10.1016/s0140-6736(82)92749-0)

[6] Schneider HJ, Dimopoulou C, Stalla GK, Reincke M, Schopohlclin J. Discriminatory value of signs and symptoms in Cushing's syndrome revisited: What has changed in 30 years? Clinical Endocrinology. 2013;**78**:152-153. DOI: 10.1111/j.1365-2265.2012.04488

[7] León-Justel A, Madrazo-Atutxa A, Alvarez-Rios AI, Infantes-Fontán R, Garcia-Arnés JA, Lillo-Muñoz JA, et al. A probabilistic model for Cushing's síndrome screening in at-risk populations: A prospective multicenter study. The Journal of Clinical Endocrinology and Metabolism. 2016;**101**:3747-3754. DOI: 10.1210/jc.2016-1673

[8] Kosilek RP, Schopohl J, Grunke M, Reincke M, Dimopoulou C, Stalla GK, et al. Automatic face classification of Cushing's Syndrome in women. A novel screening approach. Experimental and Clinical Endocrinology & Diabetes. 2013;**121**:561-564. DOI: 10.1055/s-0033-1349124

[9] Zini G. Abnormalities in leukocyte morphology and number. In: Porwit A, Mcullough J, Erber WN, editors. Blood and Bone Marrow Pathology. 2nd ed. Edinburgh: Churchill Livingstone, Elsevier; 2011. pp. 247-261

[10] Rosenfield RL. Hirsutism. The New England Journal of Medicine. 2005;**353**:2578-2588. DOI: 10.1056/NEJMcp033496

[11] Findling RH. Differentiation of pathologic/neoplastic hypercortisolism (Cushing's syndrome) from physiologic/non-neoplastic hypercortisolism (formerly known as pseudo-Cushing's Syndrome). European Journal of Endocrinology. 2017;**176**:R205-R216. DOI: 10.1530/EJE-16-0946

[12] Pecori Giraldi F, Pivonello R, Ambrogio AG, De Martino MC, De Martin M, Scacchi M, et al. The dexamethasone-suppressed corticotropin-releasing hormone stimulation test and the desmopressin test to distinguish Cushing's syndrome from pseudo-Cushing's states. Clinical Endocrinology. 2007;**66**:251-257. DOI: 10.1111/j.1365-2265.2006.02717.x

[13] Alwani RA, Schmit Jongbloed LW, de Jong FH, van der Lely AJ, de Herder WW, Feelders RA. Differentiating between Cushing's disease and pseudo-Cushing's syndrome: Comparison of four tests. European Journal of Endocrinology. 2014;**170**: 477-486. DOI: 10.1530/EJE-13-0702

[14] Castonguay TW. Glucocorticoids as modulators in the control of feeding. Brain Research Bulletin. 1991;**27**: 423-428. DOI: 10.1016/0361-9230(91) 90136-8

[15] Berthon BS, MacDonald-Wicks LK, Wood LG. A systematic review of the effect of oral glucocorticoids on energy intake, appetite, and body weight in humans. Nutrition Research. 2014;**34**: 179-190. DOI: 10.1016/j.nutres.2013. 12.006

[16] Hausman DB, Di Girolamo M, Bartness TJ, Hausman GJ, Martin RJ. The biology of white adipocyte proliferation. Obesity Reviews. 2001;**2**:239-254. DOI: 10.1046/j.1467-789x.2001.00042.x

[17] Chimin P, da Farias T, Torres-Leal FL, Bolsoni-Lopes A, Campaña AB, Andreotti S, et al. Chronic glucocorticoids treatment enhances lipogenic activity in visceral adipocytes of male Wistar rats. Acta Physiologica (Oxford, England). 2014;**211**(2): 409-420. DOI: 10.1111/apha.12226

[18] Ferrau F, Korbonits M. Metabolic comorbidities in Cushing's síndrome. European Journal of Endocrinology. 2015;**173**:M133-M157. DOI: 10.1530/EJE-15-0354

[19] Pecori Giraldi F, Moro M, Cavagnini F, Study Group on the Hypothalamo-Pituitary-Adrenal Axis of the Italian Society of Endocrinology. Gender-related differences in the presentation and course of Cushing's disease. Journal of Clinical Endocrinology Metabolism. 2003;**88**: 1554-1558. DOI: 10.1210/jc.2002-021518

[20] Drey M, Berr CM, Reincke M, Fazel J, Seissler J, Cchopohl J, et al. Beuschlein, Osswald A, Schmidmaier R Cushing's syndrome: A model for sarcopenic obesity. Endocrine. 2017; **57**:481-485. DOI: 10.1007/s12020-017-1370-x

[21] Corenblum B, Kwan T, Gee S, Wong NC. Bedside assessment of skin-fold thickness: A useful measurement for distinguishing Cushing's disease from other causes of hirsutism and oligomenorrhea. Archives of Internal Medicine. 1994;**154**:777-781. DOI: 10.1001/archinte.154.7.777

[22] Scaroni C, Zilio M, Foti M, Boscaro M. Glucose metabolism abnormalities in Cushing Syndrome: From molecular basis to clinical management. Endocrine Reviews. 2017; **38**:189-219. DOI: 10.1210/er.2016-1105

[23] Ambrogio AG, De Martin M, Ascoli P, Cavagnini F, Pecori GF. Gender-dependent changes in haematological parameters in patients with Cushing's disease before and after remission. European Journal of Endocrinology. 2014;**170**:393-400. DOI: 10.1530/EJE-13-0824

[24] Lee Y, Yi HS, Kim HR, Joung KH, Kang YE, Lee JH, et al. The eosinophil count tends to be negatively associated with levels of serum glucose in patients with adrenal Cushing Syndrome. Endocrinology and Metabolism. 2017;**32**: 353-359

[25] Broder MS, Chang E, Reddy SR, Neary MP. An approach to using data mining to support early identification of acromegaly. Endocrine Practice. 2017;**23**: 422-431. DOI: 10.4158/EP161575.OR

Chapter 4

Primary Hyperaldosteronism: The Role of the General Surgeons in Diagnosis and Treatment

Thawatchai Tullavardhana

Abstract

Primary hyperaldosteronism (PA) is the cause of endocrine hypertension, which commonly occurs in young patients with uncontrolled hypertension that leads to worsening cardiovascular-related mortality. Patients suspected of developing PA should have their plasma aldosterone concentration and plasma renin activity (PRA) assessed for screening purposes. After verifying the diagnosis of PA, adrenal venous sample (AVS) is the gold standard diagnostic technique for differentiating unilateral from bilateral disease. Since adrenalectomy may benefit patients with unilateral disease, laparoscopic adrenalectomy, a minimally invasive surgical approach that provides better postoperative outcomes than open surgery, has become the standard treatment for unilateral PA. Laparoscopic adrenalectomy resulted in a 53% cure rate of hypertension after surgery, as well as all patients had improved hypertension control, including the remission of hypokalemia. The conventional laparoscopic adrenalectomy approaches are transperitoneal and retroperitoneal, with similar postoperative outcomes. However, for general surgeons with limited laparoscopic adrenalectomy experience, the transperitoneal technique may offer an advantage over the retroperitoneal approach in terms of faster learning curve time, better surgical anatomy view, and the ability to resect adrenal tumors larger than 5 cm. This chapter focuses on the diagnosis and treatment of PA from the general surgeon's perspective.

Keywords: primary hyperaldosteronism, hypertension, adrenalectomy, minimally invasive surgery, transabdominal approach

1. Introduction

Primary hyperaldosteronism (PA) is a leading cause of endocrine hypertension attributable to the autonomous secretion of aldosterone by the adrenal gland, which inhibits the renin-angiotensin system, resulting in sodium retention, potassium diuresis, and volume overload. PA was reported as 5–11% patients with hypertension are related to 20% of drug-resistant hypertension [1–3]. In addition, patients may experience hypokalemia symptoms, such as proximal muscular weakness, muscle cramps, and palpitations. This chapter focused on the diagnosis process and the proper minimally invasive surgical treatment of PA from the general surgeon's perspective.

IntechOpen

2. Prevalence

The PA was classified into two subtypes, which are as follows: 1) unilateral adrenal gland involvement (adrenal adenoma) in 33–95% of patients, and 2) bilateral adrenal gland involvement (adrenal gland hyperplasia) in 5–60% of patients, according to certain studies. Thus, in patients with unilateral gland involvement, the goal of normalizing aldosterone levels by surgical management may be advantageous in contrast to the patients having bilateral adrenal involvement, these were more susceptible to medical treatment [4, 5].

Excessive aldosterone secretion may damage the cardiovascular system, increasing the risk of myocardial infarction, heart failure, cardiac arrhythmias (atrial fibrillation), stroke, renal function impairment, and consequences to increase cardiovascular-related mortality [6, 7].

The following were the indications for PA screening in hypertensive patients: 1) hypertension in young adults (age < 40 years), 2) severe/treatment-resistant hypertension (blood pressure > 160/100 mmHg), 3) sleep apnea, 4) hypokalemia, 5) atrial fibrillation without structural cardiac diseases, 6) first degree relative with PA, and 6) incidentaloma [8].

3. Screening test

3.1 Plasma aldosterone concentration and plasma renin activity

The plasma aldosterone concentration (PAC) is greater than 15 ng/dL, and the plasma renin activity (PRA) is less than 1 ng/mL/hour. This is the cut-off result for screening tests and was used to diagnose PA. Nonetheless, there are various methods for evaluating aldosterone levels in clinical settings, such as immunological assays and liquid chromatography-tandem MS/MS (LC–MS/MS), which may influence the cut-off values of each test.

As a result, aldosterone to renin ratio (ARR) greater than 30 ng/dL per ng/mL/h is more accepted in determining positive screening tests for PA with a sensitivity of 68–94%. To prevent a false negative result, antihypertensive medications, particularly angiotensin-converting enzyme (ACE) inhibitors and angiotensin receptor blockers (ARB), should be discontinued between 4 and 6 weeks prior to the screening is recommended [9, 10].

4. Confirmatory test

Almost all patients who had positive screening test results needed a confirmation test to access dynamic aldosterone hypersecretion that affects the imbalance of the renin-angiotensin-aldosterone system to confirm the diagnosis of PA. However, the confirmation test may not be required in patients with the following conditions: 1) PAC levels larger than 20 ng/dL and 2) spontaneous hypokalemia.

4.1 Oral sodium loading test

After achieving good blood pressure control and collecting hypokalemia, the patients were required to intake 5000 milligrams (mg) of sodium (equal to 12.8 grams of sodium chloride) for 3 days. After 3 days of the high sodium diet, 24-hour urine samples were collected for sodium and aldosterone measurements. The diagnosis of PA was confirmed by: 1) 24-hour urinary sodium excretion greater than 200 mEq, and 2) 24-hour urinary aldosterone excretion greater than 12 micrograms. The sensitivity and specificity of the oral sodium loading test for the diagnosis of PA were reported as 96% and 93%, respectively [11, 12].

4.2 Intravenous saline infusion test

In order to reduce aldosterone production, this approach involves intravenous delivery of normal saline solution (0.9% sodium chloride) at a rate of 2 liters every 4 hours following an overnight fast. For PAC assessment, a blood sample was obtained after a complete saline infusion. In normal patients, the PAC level might be decreased to less than 5 ng/dL, however, a PAC level greater than 10 ng/dL is consistent with the diagnosis of PA with high sensitivity and specificity of 87% and 94%, respectively [13].

4.3 Fludrocortisone suppression test (FST)

Patients are given 0.1 mg of fludrocortisone orally every 6 hours for 4 days, along with potassium chloride and sodium chloride (6 gram/day) supplements to maintain serum potassium level greater than 4 mmol/L and 24-hour urine sodium excretion greater than 200 mEq. Blood samples were obtained at 7 AM to assess plasma cortisol, and at 10 AM to assess PAC, PRA, and cortisol levels. The diagnosis of PA was confirmed by: 1) a PAC level greater than 6 ng/dL, 2) a PRA level less than 1 ng/mL/h, and 3) a cortisol level at 10:00 AM that was lower than at 7:00 AM. In comparison with the saline infusion test, both tests were reliable, but FST seems to be more expensive and complex in the diagnosis of PA after a positive screening test [14].

4.4 Captopril challenge test

After 1 hour of the patients remaining in a sitting or standing position, captopril 25–50 mg was administered orally. Blood samples were taken to access PAC and PRA at 0, 1, and 2 hours after the medication was administered. The diagnosis of PA was confirmed by: 1) a decrease in PAC of more than 30% at 2 hours, 2) inability to suppress PAC to less than 11 ng/dL, and 3) an ARR of 20 ng/dL per ng/mL per hour. Furthermore, an ARR greater than 30 ng/dL per ng/mL per hour after ingesting captopril is strongly indicated for the diagnosis of PA [15, 16].

5. Radiologic imaging

5.1 Computed tomography scan (CT scan)

Contrast-enhanced CT scan is the first step in radiologic imaging in a PA patient for subtype evaluation, which is useful in distinguishing unilateral adrenal adenoma from bilateral adrenal hyperplasia, particularly in tumor sizes greater than 1–2 centimeters (cm). The CT scan detected unilateral adrenal involvement with 100% accuracy in a patient under the age of 35 with hypokalemia and a PAC greater than 30 ng/dL. The accuracy rate of CT scan declined in the patients over the age of 35, which is attributed to the high prevalence of bilateral disease and the limitations of

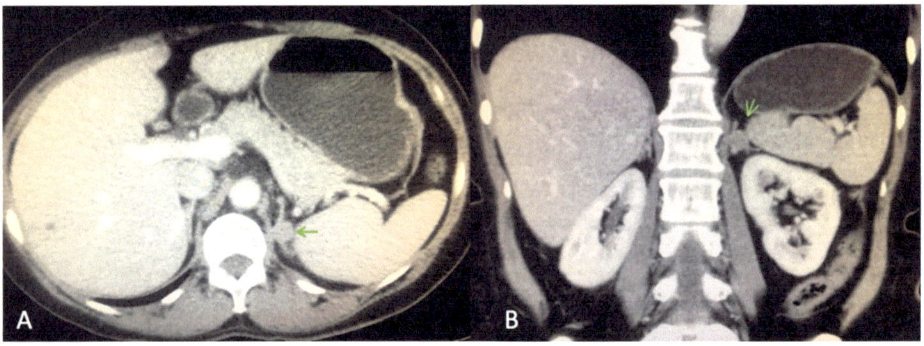

Figure 1.
Computed tomography (CT) shows a well-defined left adrenal nodule (arrow) of size 1.3 cm. (18 HF on noncontrast CT) compatible with adrenal adenoma: (A) Sagittal view, and (B) coronal view.

the CT scan in differentiating the normal appearing adrenal gland from microadenomas (size less than 1 cm).

There are no CT criteria for differentiating adenoma from bilateral adrenal hyperplasia in terms of size and Hounsfield units. Nevertheless, the study by Lingam et al., demonstrates that an adrenal limb greater than 3 millimeters is beneficial in the diagnosis of adrenal hyperplasia with 100% sensitivity and specificity [17, 18]. **Figure 1** illustrates CT scan-detected left aldosterone-producing adenoma.

5.2 Magnetic resonance imaging (MRI)

High-resolution MRI, including T1 and T2 weight images, has the same detection rate for unilateral adrenal adenoma as CT and should be used as a diagnostic adjunct in patients with strong clinical indications of PA and negative or equivocal CT findings. Furthermore, the diagnostic value of MRI for bilateral adrenal hyperplasia is limited in patients older than 40 years, with 68% sensitivity and 57% specificity [19, 20].

6. Role of lateralization with adrenal venous sampling (AVS)

Adrenal venous sampling is the gold standard diagnostic tool for differentiating unilateral from bilateral disease in PA patients. Aldosterone hypersecretion was discovered in the absence of an enlarged adrenal gland or a nodule. Thus, AVS improves the accuracy of the diagnosis of PA by 20–38% when compared to CT or MRI imaging, which can guide proper management and minimize unnecessary adrenalectomy in 20% of patients using the imaged-base technique.

The current guidelines for PA care are determined based on AVS findings. An interventional radiologist used percutaneous femoral vein access to perform this procedure. Blood samples were taken from the veins in the adrenal glands and the inferior vena cava (IVC).

The unilateral lateral disease was diagnosed when the ratio of normalized aldosterone to cortisol between the dominant and nondominant adrenal glands (lateralization index) was at least 4.0 and the ratio of aldosterone normalized to cortisol between the nondominant adrenal gland and peripheral blood (suppression ratio) was equal or less than 1.0.

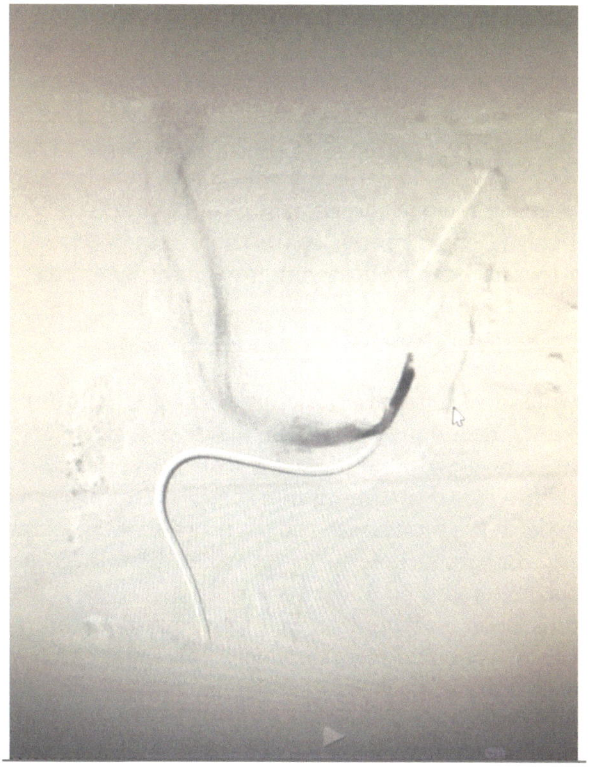

Figure 2.
Angiographic imaging of adrenal venous sampling via the left adrenal vein.

Furthermore, AVS-based decision-making was found to be superior to image-based decision-making in unilateral pathology, resulting in hypokalemia correction and improved blood pressure control with 35–60% requiring no further antihypertensive drugs [21–23]. **Figure 2** illustrates adrenal venous sampling in patients with left primary hyperaldosteronism.

7. Role of surgical management in primary hyperaldosteronism

Patients with bilateral disease were considered for medical treatment with mineralocorticoid receptor antagonists, such as spironolactone or eplerenone, in conjunction with potassium chloride supplementation. In contrast, surgical adrenalectomy may reduce aldosterone levels to normal in unilateral hyper-aldosterone-producing adenoma. Adrenalectomy can cure hypertension among 30–60% of patients and completely correct hypokalemia, resulting in a decreased incidence of atrial fibrillation and cardiovascular-related mortality in PA patients [24, 25].

7.1 Open surgery versus minimally invasive surgery

Historically, open adrenalectomy was the treatment of choice for functioning adrenal adenoma. After the development of minimally invasive surgical techniques, Gagner et al. first described laparoscopic adrenalectomy in 1992 for the management of Cushing's syndrome and pheochromocytoma [26].

Laparoscopic adrenalectomy provides an advantage over open surgery in terms of decreased intraoperative blood loss, less postoperative complications, shorter return to diet time, shorter length of hospital stays, and faster return to normal activity [27].

Laparoscopic adrenalectomy is beneficial for long-term blood pressure control and correction of hypokalemia in patients with PA. The cure rate for hypertension was 51%, with conversion to open surgery and postoperative morbidity rates of 3.2% and 8.0%, respectively [28]. Currently, laparoscopic adrenalectomy is considered the standard treatment for unilateral aldosterone-producing adenoma.

7.2 Transperitoneal versus retroperitoneal approach

The transperitoneal and retroperitoneal approaches are used for standard laparoscopic adrenalectomy techniques. The retroperitoneal technique is advantageous in cases of previous extensive abdominal surgery to avoid visceral organ injury, but it should be avoided in adrenal tumors greater than 7 cm in size, since this may limit anatomical landmarks in the retroperitoneal space. Previous research indicates that both procedures are comparable in terms of operating time, intraoperative blood loss, hospital stay, and postoperative complications [29, 30].

Attributed to the reason that the author's institution is a medium-sized university hospital, general surgeons must play an important role in the minimally invasive surgical management of patients with functional adrenal tumors, particularly pheochromocytoma and primary hyperaldosteronism.

Transperitoneal approach appears to be an appropriate surgical technique for general surgeons with limited experience in laparoscopic adrenalectomy because of 1) shorter learning curve time, 2) superior surgical view through the use of laparoscopy, 3) comfort with intraperitoneal anatomical landmarks over retroperitoneal space, and 4) ability to resect adrenal tumors larger than 5 cm. The retroperitoneal technique is appropriate for experienced surgeons who have conducted at least 20 procedures and also have a tumor size of less than 5 cm [31–32].

8. Operative techniques for laparoscopic transperitoneal adrenalectomy

8.1 Right adrenalectomy

8.1.1 Patient position

The operation was performed under general anesthesia and the patients were placed in a left lateral decubitus position, and the surgical table was flexed between 100 and 120 degrees at an umbilical level to enhance the distance between the costal margin and the iliac crest [33–36].

8.1.2 Trocars site placement

A 12 mm trocar was introduced into the peritoneal cavity using an open method at 3 cm below the right costal margin at the anterior axillary. Under laparoscopic guidance, two 5 mm working trocars were placed in the posterior axillary line and mid-clavicular line. The author preferred to add a 5 mm trocar at the subxiphoid for a fan-shaped liver retractor.

8.1.3 Operative technique

After carbon dioxide insufflation, pneumoperitoncum is created with a pressure of 10–12 mmHg. The triangular ligament was divided and the right lobe of the liver was lifted upward with a fan-shaped liver retractor. The posterior peritoneum was dissected with an electrocautery hook or harmonic scalpel (Ethicon Endo-Surgery INC - Johnson & Johnson, NJ, USA) to expose the right kidney, right adrenal gland, and inferior vena cava (IVC).

The first and most crucial step in right adrenalectomy is vascular control. Thus, the superomedial aspect of the adrenal gland, which is located between the confluence of the IVC and the right renal vein, was meticulously dissected to identify the right adrenal vein.

The right adrenal vein was clipped with nonabsorbable polymer clips (hem-o-lock(R), Teleflex Medical, Durham, NC, USA) and divided by a laparoscopic scissor or harmonic scalpel. The author recommended the use of double clips on the IVC site to avoid clip slippage, which could result in exsanguinate bleeding.

Following control of the right adrenal vein, the adrenal gland was raised up with an atraumatic grasper, and dissection should be extended to the posterior and lateral aspects to complete adrenal gland removal.

The gland is placed in a sterile bag before being retrieved via a 12 mm trocar incision that can be extended as needed. Before closing the skin incision, complete

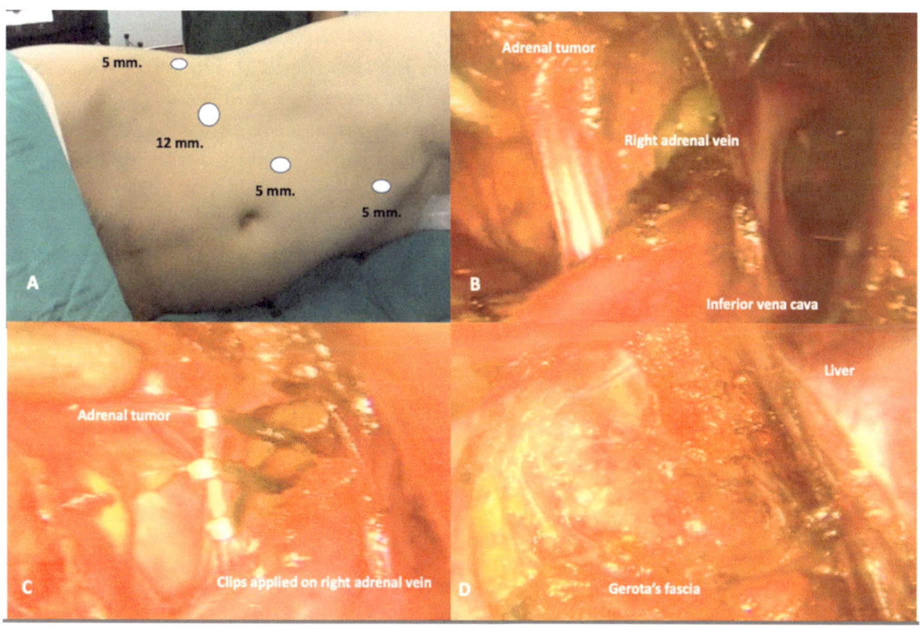

Figure 3.
Laparoscopic transperitoneal right adrenalectomy: (A) Position of the patient and placement of the trocars; (B) identification of the right adrenal vein; (C) clips control of the right adrenal vein; and (D) after removal of the right adrenal tumor.

hemostasis was confirmed, and routine drainage was not recommended. **Figure 3** illustrates the surgical technique for laparoscopic transperitoneal right adrenalectomy.

8.2 Left adrenalectomy

8.2.1 Patient position

The patients were placed in the right lateral decubitus position and the operating table was flexed, as described in right adrenalectomy.

8.2.2 Trocars site placement

An open 12 mm trocar was introduced into the peritoneal cavity 3 cm below the left costal margin at the anterior axillary line. Two 5 mm and 12 mm working trocars were placed at the subxiphoid and mid-clavicular lines, respectively. An extra 5 mm trocar can be placed in the posterior axillary line as necessary for the fan-shaped retractor.

8.2.3 Operative technique

The procedure for creating pneumoperitoneum is the same as that described in right adrenalectomy. The splenic flexure colon and spleen were mobilized initially by dissecting the splenocolic, splenorenal, and lienorenal ligaments through the diaphragm for adequate exposure of the left adrenal gland.

The upper pole of Gerota's fascia serves as a landmark for identifying the left adrenal gland during dissection. The dissection was carried out medially close to the level of the left renal vein. Meticulous dissection was required to locate the left adrenal vein, which was subsequently clipped and separated from the left renal vein using nonabsorbable polymer clips (hem-o-lock(R), Teleflex Medical, Durham, NC, USA).

The adrenal gland's medial aspect was carefully dissected, and the small arterial branches from the aorta that supply the left adrenal gland were clipped and divided. Completer gland removal was accomplished by continuing dissection to the upper portion of the gland while avoiding harm to the splenic artery and pancreatic tail. After hemostasis was confirmed, the specimen was retrieved using a sterile bag. **Figure 4** illustrates the surgical technique for laparoscopic transperitoneal left adrenalectomy.

8.3 Postoperative complication

For the right adrenalectomy, significant bleeding occurs as a result of IVC injury caused by avulsion or right adrenal vein or clip slippage, necessitating conversion to open surgery. This complication may have been avoided with proper trocar site placement and precise dissection to allow adequate exposure of the surgical landmarks via the laparoscopic view.

Left adrenalectomy complications included hollow viscus organ perforation, vascular injury, and pancreatic tail injury. These could be prevented by using the proper trocar site placement and surgical dissection technique. In the case of small adrenal tumors, the upper pole of Gerota's fascia is an essential surgical landmark for determining the appropriate dissection plane to identify the adrenal gland. This technique could prevent the dissection of the incorrect plane, thereby preventing bleeding from the renal and splenic veins.

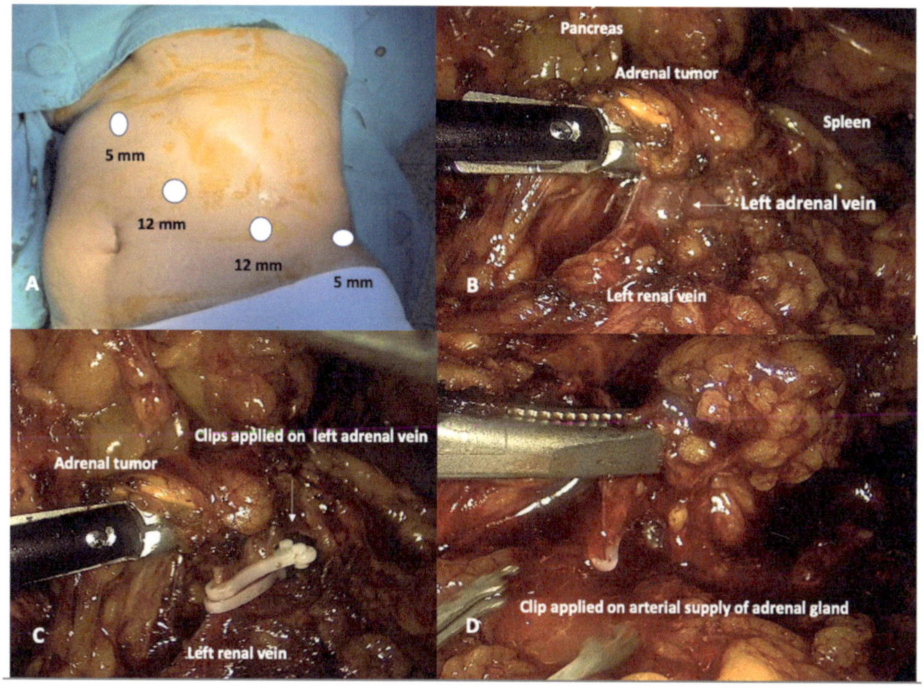

Figure 4.
Laparoscopic transperitoneal left adrenalectomy: (A) Patient positioning and trocar site placement; (B) identification of the left adrenal vein; (C) control of the left adrenal vein with clips; and (D) control of the arterial supply to the left adrenal gland with clips.

In the circumstance that renal artery or renal vein injury occurs during adrenal gland dissection. The damage site might be controlled with an atraumatic grasper and repaired with an intracorporeal suture. However, if the hemorrhage cannot be controlled, immediate conversion to open surgery will be required.

Hollow viscous organ perforation should be repaired with an intracorporal suture under laparoscopic vision, similar to pancreatic tail injury; in this circumstance, closed-suction drainage at the surgical site should be considered.

9. Postoperative disease monitoring

For immediate postoperative disease monitoring, blood tests for plasma aldosterone, renin, and potassium levels should start on the first day. Therefore, antihypertensive medications and potassium supplements should be discontinued or tapered to prevent interfering with biochemical measurements.

Furthermore, serum aldosterone and renin levels should be measured at 1 and 6 months after surgical management to confirm that PA is curable. Patients who underwent adrenalectomy under AVS-based therapy had a high biochemical cure rate of 80%, attributable to the improvement in hypertension control and hypokalemia cure rates [37, 38]. **Video 1** (https://drive.google.com/file/d/1J5Z03Kb7ZCXVOGZEWthVpEZOc-p3u3EM/view) shows a technique in laparoscopic left adrenalectomy via transperitoneal approach in a patient with primary hyperaldosteronism.

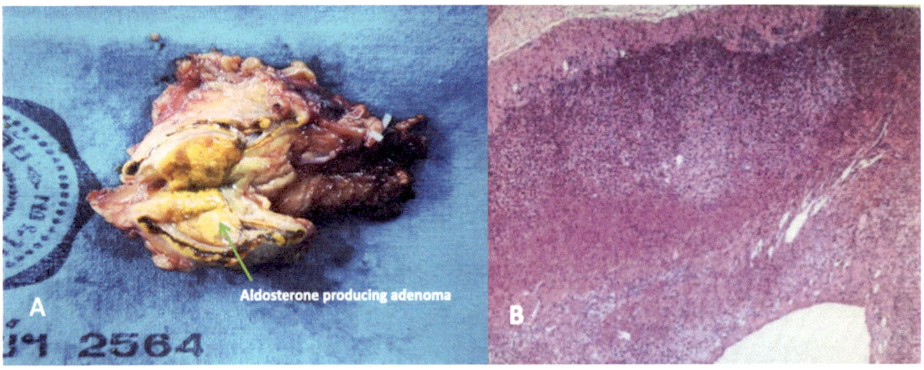

Figure 5.
Surgical specimen: (A) Gross specimen reveals 1.5 and 0.3 cm of golden yellow adrenal adenoma, and (B) microscopic examination of tumor cells reveals an alveolar and trabecular pattern of growth without capsular or vascular invasion.

The postoperative hypertension cure rate following adrenalectomy was found to be 53% at 6 months and 49.6% at 12 months. Age older than 55 years, a long history of hypertension, and a tumor size greater than 2 cm are indeed risk factors for postoperative persistent hypertension. All of the patients, however, had curative hypokalemia and needed fewer antihypertensive medications following the surgery [39–41]. **Figure 5** illustrates a surgical specimen from laparoscopic left adrenalectomy in PA patients.

10. Conclusion

Laparoscopic adrenalectomy is the gold standard treatment for unilateral PA, with a low postoperative morbidity rate and an excellent clinical success rate for hypertension control. General surgeons, particularly in small to medium-sized hospitals, may play an important role in the surgical management of PA. Transperitoneal laparoscopic adrenalectomy is a safe and effective technique that is recommended for general surgeons with limited laparoscopic adrenalectomy experience.

Acknowledgements

The author wishes to thank Associate Professor Prinya Akkranurakul for the comments, who contributed in the preparation of this chapter.

Conflict of interest

The author declared no conflict of interest.

DOI: http://dx.doi.org/10.5772/intechopen.107460

Author details

Thawatchai Tullavardhana
Department of Surgery, Faculty of Medicine, Srinakharinwirot University, Ongkharak, Nakhon Nayok, Thailand

*Address all correspondence to: thawatchait@g.swu.ac.th

References

[1] Reincke M, Bancos I, Mulatero P, Scholl UI, Stowasser M, Williams TA. Diagnosis and treatment of primary aldosteronism. The Lancet Diabetes and Endocrinology. 2021;**9**(12):876-892

[2] Hundemer GL, Vaidya A. Primary aldosteronism diagnosis and management: A clinical approach. Endocrinology and Metabolism Clinics of North America. 2019;**48**(4):681-700

[3] Douma S, Petidis K, Doumas M, Papaefthimiou P, Triantafyllou A, Kartali N, et al. Prevalence of primary hyperaldosteronism in resistant hypertension: A retrospective observational study. Lancet. 2008;**371**(9628):1921-1926

[4] Iacobone M, Citton M, Viel G, Rossi GP, Nitti D. Approach to the surgical management of primary aldosteronism. Gland Surgery. 2015;**4**(1):69-81

[5] Fagugli RM, Taglioni C. Changes in the perceived epidemiology of primary hyperaldosteronism. International Journal of Hypertension. 2011;**2011**:162804

[6] Monticone S, D'Ascenzo F, Moretti C, Williams TA, Veglio F, Gaita F, et al. Cardiovascular events and target organ damage in primary aldosteronism compared with essential hypertension: A systematic review and meta-analysis. The Lancet Diabetes and Endocrinology. 2018;**6**(1):41-50

[7] Reincke M, Fischer E, Gerum S, Merkle K, Schulz S, Pallauf A, et al. German Conn's registry-else kröner-fresenius-hyperaldosteronism registry. Observational study mortality in treated primary aldosteronism: The German Conn's registry. Hypertension. 2012;**60**(3):618-624

[8] Vaidya A, Carey RM. Evolution of the primary aldosteronism syndrome: Updating the approach. The Journal of Clinical Endocrinology and Metabolism. 2020;**105**(12):3771-3783

[9] Funder JW, Carey RM, Mantero F, Murad MH, Reincke M, Shibata H, et al. Themanagementofprimaryaldosteronism: Case detection, diagnosis, and treatment: An endocrine society clinical practice guideline. The Journal of Clinical Endocrinology and Metabolism. 2016;**101**(5):1889-1916

[10] Young WF Jr. Diagnosis and treatment of primary aldosteronism: Practical clinical perspectives. Journal of Internal Medicine. 2019;**285**(2):126-148

[11] Morera J, Reznik Y. Management of endocrine disease: The role of confirmatory tests in the diagnosis of primary aldosteronism. European Journal of Endocrinology. 2019;**180**(2):R45-R58

[12] Bravo EL, Tarazi RC, Dustan HP, Fouad FM, Textor SC, Gifford RW, et al. The changing clinical spectrum of primary aldosteronism. The American Journal of Medicine. 1983;**74**(4):641-651

[13] Stowasser M, Ahmed AH, Cowley D, Wolley M, Guo Z, McWhinney BC, et al. Comparison of seated with recumbent saline suppression testing for the diagnosis of primary aldosteronism. The Journal of Clinical Endocrinology and Metabolism. 2018;**103**(11):4113-4124

[14] Mulatero P, Milan A, Fallo F, Regolisti G, Pizzolo F, Fardella C, et al. Comparison of confirmatory tests for the diagnosis of primary aldosteronism. The

Journal of Clinical Endocrinology and Metabolism. 2006;**91**(7):2618-2623

[15] Giacchetti G, Ronconi V, Lucarelli G, Boscaro M, Mantero F. Analysis of screening and confirmatory tests in the diagnosis of primary aldosteronism: Need for a standardized protocol. Journal of Hypertension. 2006;**24**(4):737-745

[16] Kidoguchi S, Sugano N, Hayashi-Ishikawa N, Morisawa N, Tokudome G, Yokoo T. The characteristics of captopril challenge test-positive patients using various criteria. Journal of the Renin-Angiotensin-Aldosterone System. 2019;**20**(3):170

[17] Lee SH, Kim JW, Yoon HK, Koh JM, Shin CS, Kim SW, et al. Diagnostic accuracy of computed tomography in predicting primary aldosteronism subtype according to age. Endocrinol Metab (Seoul). 2021;**36**(2):401-412

[18] Lingam RK, Sohaib SA, Vlahos I, Rockall AG, Isidori AM, Monson JP, et al. CT of primary hyperaldosteronism (Conn's syndrome): The value of measuring the adrenal gland. AJR. American Journal of Roentgenology. 2003;**181**(3):843-849

[19] Wang JH, Wu HM, Sheu MH, Tseng HS, Chiang JH, Chang CY. High resolution MRI of adrenal glands in patients with primary aldosteronism. Zhonghua Yi Xue Za Zhi (Taipei). 2000;**63**(6):475-481

[20] Zhou Y, Wang D, Jiang L, Ran F, Chen S, Zhou P, et al. Diagnostic accuracy of adrenal imaging for subtype diagnosis in primary aldosteronism: Systematic review and meta-analysis. BMJ Open. 2020;**10**:e038489

[21] Kempers MJ, Lenders JW, van Outheusden L, van der Wilt GJ, Schultze Kool LJ, Hermus AR, et al. Systematic review: Diagnostic procedures to differentiate unilateral from bilateral adrenal abnormality in primary aldosteronism. Annals of Internal Medicine. 2009;**151**(5):329-337

[22] Dekkers T, Prejbisz A, Kool LJS, Groenewoud HJMM, Velema M, Spiering W, et al. Adrenal vein sampling versus CT scan to determine treatment in primary aldosteronism: An outcome-based randomized diagnostic trial. The Lancet Diabetes and Endocrinology. 2016;**4**(9):739-746

[23] Fingeret AL, Lee JA. Adrenal venous sampling in primary hyperaldosteronism. Current Surgery Reports. 2014;**2**:38

[24] Hundemer GL, Vaidya A. Management of endocrine disease: The role of surgical adrenalectomy in primary aldosteronism. European Journal of Endocrinology. 2020;**183**(6):R185-R196

[25] Jing Y, Liao K, Li R, Yang S, Song Y, He W, et al. Cardiovascular events and all-cause mortality in surgically or medically treated primary aldosteronism: A meta-analysis. Journal of the Renin-Angiotensin-Aldosterone System. 2021;**22**(1):1470

[26] Gagner M, Lacroix A, Bolté E. Laparoscopic adrenalectomy in Cushing's syndrome and pheochromocytoma. The New England Journal of Medicine. 1992;**327**(14):1033

[27] Li J, Wang Y, Chang X, Han Z. Laparoscopic adrenalectomy (LA) vs. open adrenalectomy (OA) for pheochromocytoma (PHEO): A systematic review and meta-analysis. European Journal of Surgical Oncology. 2020;**46**(6):991-998

[28] Pang TC, Bambach C, Monaghan JC, Sidhu SB, Bune A, Delbridge LW, et al.

Outcomes of laparoscopic adrenalectomy for hyperaldosteronism. ANZ Journal of Surgery. 2007;**77**(9):768-773

[29] Rubinstein M, Gill IS, Aron M, Kilciler M, Meraney AM, Finelli A, et al. Prospective, randomized comparison of transperitoneal versus retroperitoneal laparoscopic adrenalectomy. The Journal of Urology. 2005;**174**(2):442-445

[30] Nigri G, Rosman AS, Petrucciani N, Fancellu A, Pisano A, Zorcolo L, et al. Meta-analysis of trials comparing laparoscopic transperitoneal and retroperitoneal adrenalectomy. Surgery. 2013;**153**(1):111-119

[31] Liu Z, Li DW, Yan L, Xu ZH, Gu GL. Comparison of lateral transperitoneal and retroperitoneal approaches for homolateral laparoscopic adrenalectomy. BMC Surgery. 2021;**21**(1):432

[32] Ottlakan A, Paszt A, Simonka Z, Abraham S, Borda B, Vas M, et al. Laparoscopic transperitoneal and retroperitoneal adrenalectomy: A 20-year, single-institution experience with an analysis of the learning curve and tumor size. Surgical Endoscopy. 2020;**34**(12):5421-5427

[33] Tullavardhana T. Laparoscopic adrenalectomy: Surgical technique. WJOLS. 2010;**3**(2):91-97

[34] Di Buono G, Buscemi S, Lo Monte AI, Geraci G, Sorce V, Citarrella R, et al. Laparoscopic adrenalectomy: Preoperative data, surgical technique and clinical outcomes. BMC Surgery. 2019;**18**(Suppl. 1):128

[35] Uludağ M, Aygün N, İşgör A. Surgical indication and technique for adrenalectomy. Med Bull Sisli Etfal Hosp. 2020;**54**(1):8-22

[36] Kwak J, Lee KE. Minimally invasive adrenal surgery. Endocrinol Metab (Seoul). 2020;**35**(4):774-783

[37] Rossi GP, Cesari M, Lenzini L, Seccia TM. Disease monitoring of primary aldosteronism. Best Practice & Research. Clinical Endocrinology & Metabolism. 2020;**34**(2):101417

[38] Thiesmeyer JW, Ullmann TM, Stamatiou AT, Limberg J, Stefanova D, Beninato T, et al. Association of adrenal venous sampling with outcomes in primary aldosteronism for unilateral adenomas. JAMA Surgery. **156**(2):165-171

[39] Zhou Y, Zhang M, Ke S, Liu L. Hypertension outcomes of adrenalectomy in patients with primary aldosteronism: A systematic review and meta-analysis. BMC Endocrine Disorders. 2017;**17**(1):61

[40] Carter Y, Roy M, Sippel RS, Chen H. Persistent hypertension after adrenalectomy for an aldosterone-producing adenoma: Weight as a critical prognostic factor for aldosterone's lasting effect on the cardiac and vascular systems. The Journal of Surgical Research. 2012;**177**(2):241-247

[41] Goh BK, Tan YH, Yip SK, Eng PH, Cheng CW. Outcome of patients undergoing laparoscopic adrenalectomy for primary hyperaldosteronism. Journal of the Society of Laparoendoscopic. 2004;**8**(4):320-325

Chapter 5

Congenital Adrenal Hyperplasia

Adina Mariana Ghemigian and Nicoleta Dumitru

Abstract

Congenital adrenal hyperplasia (CAH) is a rare pathology with an estimated incidence of 1:14,000–18,000 births. It includes a group of inherited diseases with autosomal recessive transmission. The genetic defect consists of mutations of the genes encoding the enzymes involved in adrenal and eventually gonadal steroidogenesis. The most common mutation is the gene encoding 21 hydroxylase the enzyme involved in cortisol and aldosterone synthesis. However, other enzymatic defects can be identified. The excess of steroid precursors in the adrenal cortex will be directed towards adrenal androgen synthesis. Finally, the clinical picture includes a series of manifestations specific to the enzymatic deficiency, the severity depending on the degree of the genetic defect. Thus, we can meet severe deficits with clinical expression in newborns and toddlers or partial, non-classical forms with manifestation in adolescence or adulthood. Once the diagnosis of CAH is established, patients will require specific therapy and long-term monitoring.

Keywords: congenital adrenal hyperplasia, adrenal steroid synthesis, 21-hydroxylase deficiency, hyperandrogenism, dexamethasone

1. Introduction

Congenital adrenal hyperplasia (CAH) includes a heterogeneous group of autosomal recessive disorders caused by total or partial impairment of steroidogenesis, which is characterized by decreased synthesis of cortisol and, or aldosterone [1]. Cortisol deficiency causes an increase in ACTH levels by losing the effect of negative feedback on the hypothalamic-pituitary region. In turns this leads to chronic overstimulation of the adrenal cortex and consecutive adrenal hyperplasia.

From the point of view of steroid synthesis, the adrenal cortex is divided into three areas: zona glomerulosa or the outer layer, the site of mineralocorticoid synthesis, the fasciculata area, the middle largest layer, the site of glucocorticoid synthesis and the inner layer or zona reticularis involved in androgen biosynthesis [1]. Steroidogenesis involves the conversion of cholesterol to active steroid hormones and is performed under the action of many enzymes, cofactors, and accessory proteins (**Figure 1**) [1]. These enzymes are specific expressed in the three areas of the adrenal cortex, depending on the type of steroids synthesized, but some are also expressed in the gonads or placenta.

The pathophysiological mechanism of CAH consists in mutations in most of the genes encoding the enzymes involved in adrenal and eventually gonadal steroidogenesis. Impaired enzyme function in a specific step of adrenal steroid biosynthesis leads to a unique combination of elevated precursors and deficient products [2]. For this

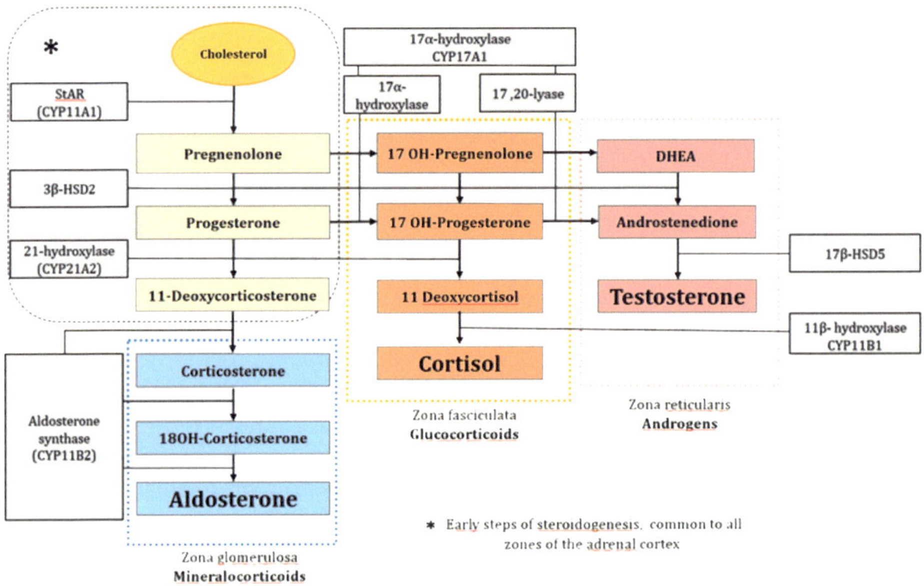

Figure 1.
Enzymatic steps of adrenal steroid synthesis.

reason, the clinical phenotype is variable and depends on the severity of the enzyme deficiency. The most common enzyme deficiency that disrupt cortisol synthesis leading to CAH is that of 21 hydroxylase [1–4].

2. 21-hydroxylase deficiency

2.1 Epidemiology

CAH due to 21-hydroxylase deficiency (21OHD) represents approximately 90–95% of CAH cases encountered in clinical practice [3, 4].

Depending on the degree of enzyme deficiency, it is classified into classical and non-classical form. Classical form occurs in 1:14,000 to 1:18,000 live births based on screening programs [1, 4, 5]. Non-classical form is more common with a prevalence of 1:500 to 1:1000 in the general white population [4]. In certain population groups like the Ashkenazi Jewish the prevalence is even higher with 1 in 27 individuals affected and 1 in 3 are carriers of the allele, making this form the most frequent autosomal recessive disorder in population [2].

2.2 Pathophysiology

CYP21A2 is a microsomal enzyme belonging to the cytochrome P450 family, also known as P450c21 [1]. The major substrate of CYP21A2 is 17 hydroxyprogesterone (17OHP), which is converted to 11-deoxycortisol in zona fasciculata, an intermediate metabolite in the cortisol synthesis stage. In zona glomerulosa, CYP21A2 acts on progesterone, converting it to 11-deoxycorticosterone within the aldosterone pathway [1]. Blocking this enzymatic step will cause cortisol deficiency with a secondary increase in ACTH secretion [2]. This in turn, will stimulate excessive synthesis of precursor molecules in both pathways blocked by the enzyme deficiency, namely 17OHP and progesterone. The precursor will be redirected to adrenal androgens synthesis via the 17,20-lyase activity of CYP17A1, the step unaffected by the enzyme deficiency [1, 2].

Intrauterine exposure to excess adrenal androgens will not significantly influence male sexual differentiation. The situation is totally different in the case of a fetus 46, XX. In this case, excess of androgens will interfere with the differentiation of the external genitalia, causing prenatal virilization. The severity of virilization is quantified using a five-point scale developed by Prader, where grade I involves minimal virilization with clitoral hypertrophy, while grade V is a typical male aspect of the external genitalia [2].

2.3 Genetics

The gene that encodes CYP21A2 is located on the short arm of the 6 chromosomes within the HLA class III region (6p21.3) arranged in tandem with its inactive pseudogene (*CYP21A1P*) [1, 3]. Both *CYP21A2* and *CYP21A1P* genes share a high nucleotide homology of about 98% and 96% in exons and introns respectively, but only *CYP21A2* gene encodes the active microsomal P450 enzyme, 21-hydroxylase (CYP21A2, P450c21) [1, 6]. The pseudogene CYP21A1P is inactive because of the presence of multiple pathogenic variants, small insertions or deletions and point pathogenic variants that prevent the synthesis of a functional protein [3, 7].

In about 70–75% of cases *CYP21A2* mutations arise from gene microconversion, namely transfer of deleterious mutations from *CYP21A1P* during meiosis, generating point mutations with consecutive reduction of the enzymatic activity of CYP21A2 [1, 6]. In 20–25% of the cases, *CYP21A2* mutations are due to gross misalignment owing to unequal crossing over during meiosis leading to gene deletions, gene duplications or the appearing of a hybrid gene or pseudogene-gene chimeras, yielding a non-functional *CYP21A2* gene [3, 6]. Less than 5% of the pathogenic variants in the CYP21A2 gene are de novo point mutations, most of these affected patients are heterozygous [3, 6].

2.4 Genotype-t correlation

Most patients with 21OHD are heterozygous compounds, with more than one mutation in one or both *CYP21A2* alleles, which is why there is a wide spectrum of phenotypes [1, 4]. In general, the phenotype reflects the residual activity of the lightest mutation [3, 7].

Scholastically, two forms of this condition are described, namely the classical and non-classical form. In turn, the classic form is subdivided into salt-wasting (SW) and simple virilizing (SV) form [1, 4].

The SW form is characterized by mutations in both alleles leading to complete loss of enzymatic activity, such as deletions, large gene conversions, nonsense mutations, frameshifts, and missense mutations [1].

The SV form occurs by mutation associated with complete loss of function on one allele and on the other allele a mutation that reduces enzymatic activity by 1–5%, like a nonconservative amino acid substitution, p.Ile172Asn (I172N) or splicing mutation on intron 2 [1, 4]. This mutation that alters splicing of intron 2 is particularly common in SV patients, but also in SW ones.

In the nonclassical (NC) form, most of the affected individuals are compound heterozygotes, with various mutations on each of the two alleles, of which at least one can allow enzymatic activity of 20–50% [6]. The genetic defect may be a point mutation in exon 7 (p.Val281Leu), or a missense mutation as p.Pro30Leu (P30L) [1, 4, 6]. However the clinical observations suggest that patients carrying the P30L allele are somewhat more symptomatic, being rather a borderline form between SV and NC [1].

Although we still use this classification of CAH forms, in practice we must consider the *CYP21A2* allelic variants with their phenotypic manifestations as a continuum clinical spectrum.

2.5 Clinical picture

The classic form of CAH due to 21OHD is identified in 1 of 14,000–18,000 newborns and includes the two variants: salt-wasting and simple virilizing form [1, 4].

2.5.1 Classic salt-wasting 21-OHD CAH

Of the two variants, the SW form is the most severe, but also the most common, representing about 75% of all cases [6]. It is characterized by null or minimal enzymatic activity (<1%) in both *CYP21A2* alleles, resulting in severe cortisol and aldosterone deficiency and elevated androgen levels [1, 3]. Clinically it is characterized by prenatal virilization of female girls by exposure to potent androgens (testosterone and Δ4-androstenedione) at critical stages of sexual development [6]. Aldosterone deficiency will be manifested soon after birth by the appearance of hypovolemia with hyperreninemia, hyponatremia and hyperkalemia, which associated with hypoglycemia due to severe cortisol deficiency, will generate an increased risk of seizures in these infants [2]. Also, these children are at high risk for adrenal crisis, that can occur at 1–6 weeks after birth, with azotemia, vascular collapse, shock, and finally death [6]. Affected males are more prone for a salt-wasting adrenal crisis at home because their normal male genitalia do not raise the suspicion for this condition, being discharged from the hospital without diagnosis [4, 6]. The episodes of salt loss in the infant period are similar in symptoms to pyloric stenosis or gastroenteritis with poor feeding, weight loss, failure to thrive, vomiting, dehydration [6]. The differentiation from the latter is achieved by the fact that children with CAH maintain diuresis.

2.5.2 Classic simple virilizing 21-OHD CAH

This second variant of classic CAH represents about 25 of the cases and is characterized by a reduced enzymatic activity of only 1–5%, which generates a clinical picture in which the exposure to excess androgens predominates. These children do not have episodes of salt loss due to the relatively normal production of aldosterone, but they do associate cortisol deficiency. In utero exposure of females to adrenal androgen excess results in external genital virilization at birth with varying degrees of clitoris enlargement, fusion of the labioscrotal folds, and formation of a urogenital sinus [6]. Excess androgens are imperceptible at birth in males. It should be noted that it is difficult to make a difference between SV and SW form based on the degree of virilization of an affected female at birth [6]. This is why all infants detected with classic CAH will be treated with glucocorticoid and mineralocorticoid treatment at least within the first year of life, because infants have a relative renal tubular resistance to the salt-retaining effects of aldosterone and a low sodium content diet [1].

Postnatal, both females and male's infants with SV CAH develop signs of androgen excess including precocious development of pubic and axillary hair, acne, seborrhea, comedones, acceleration of linear growth, advanced bone maturation leading to short final stature, with a consecutive catecholamine deficient secretion [6]. The pubertal development of untreated children consists:

- isosexual early pseudo-puberty in boys with disharmony between testicular development (prepubertal type) and penile enlargement (pubertal type)
- heterosexual early pseudo-puberty in girls

Persistence of glucocorticoid deficiency in adulthood may lead to impaired vascular tone and cardiac function, as a result of impaired development and function of adrenal medulla [6].

2.5.3 Non-classic 21-OHD CAH

As mentioned above, the genetic defect associated with NC form of CAH retains an enzymatic activity of 20–50% for CYP21A2. Thus, cortisol production is sufficient for a normal lifestyle, but insufficient to adequately suppress ACTH synthesis, and so the excessive androgen secretion is maintained. External genitalia are normal at birth, as are 17-hydroxyprogesterone levels, which is why these cases are not detected in neonatal screening [2, 7]. This form is usually diagnosed later during childhood or adolescence or even in adulthood, therefore in the past it was called the "late-onset" form [6, 7].

The clinical features of androgen excess are related to age at diagnosis [7]. In the case of prepubertal children, both sexes show accelerated growth, with advanced skeletal maturation compared to chronological age, premature development of pubic hair with a prevalence up to 30%, described even at the age of 6 months [2, 7]. Girls may have clitoromegaly, and boys may have enlarged penis with prepubertal testicles, similar to classic SV form [6]. In 30–60% of cases the ACTH 1–24 test reveals a slight cortisol deficiency, requiring replacement therapy during periods of stress.

In adolescents and adult women, the signs of hyperandrogenism predominate with treatment-resistant nodulo-cystic acne, seborrhea, androgenic alopecia, hirsutism, risk of infertility, increased rate of miscarriages [2, 6, 7]. Clinically they may associate a profile like polycystic ovary syndrome (PCOS) [7]. Up to 30% of women with PCOS have undiagnosed NCCAH [6].

Affected men are often asymptomatic. In their case, the diagnosis is made either from an affected female member or in the context of evaluation for peripubertal gynecomastia, short stature, infertility, oligospermia, or adrenal incidentalomas [2]. Up to 3% of adult men with bilateral adrenal events may have undiagnosed NCCAH [6].

2.6 Diagnosis

Diagnosis of CAH must be suspected in infants born with ambiguous genitalia [2]. CAH is a life-threatening disorder for this reason it is important to establish the diagnosis as early as possible.

2.6.1 Hormonal evaluation

Diagnosis of 21-OHD CAH can be confirmed biochemically by identifying high values of 17-OHP in a blood sample. Such hormonal evaluation is the basis of the newborn-screening program developed to identify affected patients with classical form of CAH [2]. This neonatal program screening is currently being used in more than 30 countries around the world to prevent morbidity and mortality from adrenal crisis [1, 4]. The screening procedure implies collection of blood samples by heel puncture at more than 24 h after birth, but not later than 1 week [8]. Clinical guidelines recommend as first-tier screens the use of immunoassays to measure 17OHP in dried blood spots, on the same filter paper cards used for other newborn screening tests [4].

A value of 17OHP on the 3rd day of life less than 30 nmol/L or 10 ng/mL is considered normal. However, there are no universally accepted standards for stratifying infants, most laboratories use a series of birth weight-adjusted cut-offs [4]. It should be noted that neonatal screening:

- has a risk of false positive results, ranging from 0.02 to 1.2%. This situation includes the samples collected less than 36 h after birth, premature, sick or stressed infants, a late maturation of 11 hydroxylase or in case of cross-reaction with sulphated metabolites and immature adrenal precursors [4, 8].

- In case of borderline first-tier test results some screening programs recommend repeating screening, reevaluating samples with a second-tier test by liquid chromatography–tandem mass spectrometry (LC-MS/MS) or perform molecular testing to identify the pathogenic variants in *CYP21A2* [3, 4, 6].

- 17OHP assay does not identify children with NC form of 21-OHD

- Direct biochemical analysis of 17OHP or other steroids using LC-MS/MS improve the positive predictive value of CAH screening. According to the current guidelines, the improvement of the screening prognosis can also be achieved through: [4].

- Measuring additional analytes: 21-deoxycortisol, produced by 11b-hydroxylation of 17OHP, is normally low even in preterm infants. Finding an elevated levels is highly specific for 21OHD.

- Measuring ratios of analytes: the sum of 17OHP and 21-deoxycortisol levels divided by the cortisol level detect all affected children with no false positives results and with a positive predictive value of 100%

- Measuring urinary metabolites: pregnantriol and 17b-hydroxypregnanolone, the 17OHP metabolites or pregnanetriolone, the 21-deoxycortisol metabolite; these metabolites are increased in CAH and have a good specificity, even in preterm infants. 17-hydroxypregnanolone is an intermediate product in the alternative or "backdoor" pathway of dihydrotestosterone synthesis [1]. This alternative pathway is a major contributor to fetal female virilization in 21OHD [1].

For infants with positive newborn screening for CAH the guidelines recommend referral to pediatric endocrinologists and evaluation by cosyntropin stimulation test [4].

When CAH is suspected later in childhood or in an adult, diagnosis confirmation is based on an early morning 17OHP [7]. After the newborn period, a morning 17OHP value below 2.5 nmol/L (or 0.8 ng/mL) in children, respectively below 6 nmol/L (or 2 ng/mL) in adults excludes the diagnosis of CAH (**Table 1**) [7]. It should be noted

17OHP values	Classic CAH	Non-classic CAH	Non-CAH
Basal	>300 nmol/L (>100 ng/mL)	>15 nmol/L (>5 ng/mL)	<6 nmol/L (<2 ng/mL)
ACTH-stimulated	>300 nmol/L (>100 ng/mL)	>30 nmol/L (>10 ng/mL)	<30 nmol/L (<10 ng/mL)

Table 1.
The basal and ACTH stimulated 17OHP levels.

that 17OHP has a pulsating secretion so, the values obtained mid-morning or in the afternoon may be normal. For this reason, it is recommended that blood be collected in the morning, 7.30–8.30 AM. In addition, in women it should be measured in the follicular phase of the menstrual cycle or in amenorrhea [7]. It should be noted that a simple determination of 17OHP may be accompanied by a false negative result, estimated at 2–11%, especially in adults with NC form [7].

The same as in the case of classic form, improving screening for NC CAH form can be achieved through 17OHP measurement by LC-MS/MS. This method provides increased analytical specificity, the ability for multiplex analysis (simultaneously measure multiple analytes like androstenedione, testosterone, 21-deoxycortisol), and the advantage of using minute specimen volumes [4].

2.6.2 Additional tests

If the clinical suspicion remains despite the use of LC-MS/MS, the next diagnostic step is the ACTH stimulation test, which is the golden standard for the diagnosis [2, 6, 7]. The ACTH stimulation test is performed in the morning, 8.00–9.00 AM. It involves administration of an intravenous injection of 250 μg of synthetic ACTH (Cosyntropinum, Cortrosyn), or 36 μg/kg in children under 1 year, with measuring the levels of 17OHP, androstenedione and cortisol at baseline and 60 min after the injection (**Table 1**).

Given the fact that in girls and women with non-classical form of CAH, the features of hyperandrogenism predominate in the clinical picture, it is important to be able to differentiate the etiology of this virilization syndrome. Thus, we can use the long dexamethasone test, with administration of dexamethasone for 4 days at a dose of:

- 1 mg/sqm/day divided into 4 doses (at 6 hours)—in children
- 2 mg/day divided into 4 doses (every 6 hours)—for adults

In CAH, in contrast to PCOS or Cushing syndrome there will be a suppression of androgen values (DHEAS, 17 (OH) P, testosterone) with minimum of 50 (75%) of the basic values, and also for cortisol level.

2.6.3 Molecular genetic testing

Molecular testing can detect CYP21A2 mutations and should be carried out in equivocal cases to support the diagnosis, for genetic counseling and for better prognostic and treatment guidance [2, 4, 7]. There are commercial kits that detect the most common 10–12 mutations. Testing should be performed in parents to confirm the parental origin of each mutation, to rule out the coexistence of two mutations on the same allele (cis), to determine compound heterozygosity, distinguish hemizygosity from homozygosity in the index case, and estimate the recurrence risk [1]. Once the *CYP21A2* pathogenic variants have been identified in an affected family member, molecular genetic prenatal testing for 21-OHD CAH can be performed [6]. Most often prenatal testing is considered when the parents have a previous child with 21OHD [1].

There are two methods used: chorionic villus biopsy and amniocentesis, implying invasive sampling [1]. By chorionic villus biopsy is obtained fetal DNA at gestational week 9–11. Amniocentesis was the initial method available for prenatal diagnosis [1]. It allows analysis of fetal hormones in amniotic fluid and can be performed at gestational week 12–14 [1]. Both methods imply an increased risk of fetal loss and do not totally allow avoiding prenatal treatment in male fetuses as they cannot be performed earlier than week 9 of gestation [1, 3].

However, noninvasive prenatal diagnostic method has been developed, which prevent prenatal treatment of males and unaffected females [5]. This method is based on PCR amplification of cell-free fetal DNA that can be isolated from maternal plasma as early as week 6–9 [1]. Protocols must include screening for Y chromosomal DNA in maternal blood, by detecting SRY gene [3]. Sequencing of cell-free fetal DNA can ascertain *CYP21A2* mutations, but not suitable in clinical settings [1, 3]. Instead, it can identify single nucleotide polymorphisms flanking CYP21A2 that are specific for the mother, father, and proband, determining the maternal and paternal alleles inherited by the fetus [1].

2.7 Management of 21OHD CAH forms

Treatment goals [1, 4]:

- preventing prenatal virilization of external genitalia in girls
- prevention of adrenal crisis and virilization
- ensuring normal growth and development
- ensuring normal pubertal maturation from birth to adolescence,
- prevention of long-term complications
- Therapeutic options:

2.7.1 Prenatal treatment

The prenatal treatment involves the use of dexamethasone in dose of 20 μg/kg/day, to maximum 1.5 mg/day given in three doses to pregnant women with a fetus at risk for classic CAH [1]. Dexamethasone has increased half-life, crosses the barrier placenta and is not degraded by placental 11βhydroxysteroid dehydrogenase type 2 (HSD11B2). It can reduce the fetal ACTH and subsequently the androgen levels, with the aim of preventing prenatal virilization of external genitalia in affected girls. The effectiveness of prenatal therapy with dexamethasone depends on when treatment is started, optimum by gestational week 6–7. The benefit is reduced to 15% in case of late initiation, early discontinuation, or reduced compliance with therapy, thus allowing slight virilization of the fetus. The treatment is controversial due to safety concerns related to exposure to dexamethasone in this stage of embryonic development that may impact much more than the hypothalamic-pituitary-adrenal axis [1].

2.7.2 Treatment of classic 21OHD CAH forms

In SW form:

- Dietary supplementation with NaCl, especially in the first months of life. The dose in breast-fed infants is 10–12 mmol/KgC/day [5].

- Mineralocorticoid replacement with fludrocortisone typically 100–200 μg/day divided in 1 or 2 oral doses, of which one must be in the morning [2, 5].

Due to relative mineralocorticoid resistance at this age and secondary to the antimineralocorticoid effects of elevated 17OHP, neonates and young infants require higher fludrocortisone doses [1]. However, the need for fludrocortisone diminishes with time. The monitoring will be done by electrolytes, plasma renin, and blood pressure measurement [2].

- Glucocorticoid replacement with hydrocortisone is the preferred option, because of its shorter half-life that minimizes the adverse side effects [1].

The hydrocortisone tablets are crushed and mixed into food or suspended and given in a dose of 10–15 mg/sqm daily, in 3–4 divided doses [1]. Treatment will be monitored every 3 months in infant younger than 18 months and every 4–6 months in older children, or more frequently after a change in dosing [1, 4]. Serum levels of 17OHP and androstenedione will be monitored. The suggested target for 17OHP level is 2–3 times the upper normal level, but not higher than 10 ng/mL (or 30 nmol/L) when measured in the early morning before medication [1]. It is recommended to avoid the normalization of the 17OHP level because of the risk of glucocorticoid overdosing causing iatrogenic Cushing syndrome [1, 2, 4].

The hydrocortisone dose may need to be dubled in case of minor intercurrences with fever below 39 degrees or tripled in case of fever above 39 degrees. Raising the dose is not recommended for everyday mental and emotional stress, minor illness, or before routine exercise [1, 4].

As growth cartilage closes, teens and later adults may receive slow-release corticosteroids, such as prednisone 5–7.5 mg/day or dexamethasone 0.25–0.5 mg/day at bedtime. However, in adults hydrocortisone remains the preferred option for glucocorticoid treatment due to its better metabolic, cardiovascular and bone mineral density outcome compare to dexamethasone or prednisone [1, 4].

Adolescents and women with clinical and ultrasound criteria for PCOS may benefit from treatment with oral contraceptives that may be associated, or not with antiandrogens (spironolactone) [4].

In SV form:

Treatment includes hydrocortisone at a dose of 8–15 mg/sqm, doses being increased in conditions of overload, except for intense physical effort [1, 4].

Replacement with mineralocorticoids is done only during infancy to allow the use of minimum doses of glucocorticoids. After this period the child will receive mineralocorticoids only if the renin values are increased [1].

A multidisciplinary team is needed in approaching the individual with genital ambiguity consisting of specialists in pediatric endocrinology, pediatric urology/surgery, clinical genetics, and psychology is essential for the best diagnosis and management [6].

Genitoplasty surgery in girls involves clitoroplasty, opening of the vaginal introitus and labioplasty [1]. Surgical techniques are intended for erectile tissue removal, keeping the clitoris with sensitive innervation, ensuring a proper vaginal opening, preventing recurrent urinary tract infections [1].

2.7.3 Treatment of non-classic 21OHD CAH form

Decisions about starting treatment should be individualized and based on clinical symptoms [2]. The guidelines do not recommend routine treatment with glucocorticoid in asymptomatic individuals [1, 4]. The main goal in children with NC CAH is to maintain normal growth and pubertal development. This childrens will be regularly monitored clinically for height, weight, signs of androgen excess, puberty, and bone age advancement [7].

Hydrocortisone treatment will be recommended in case of:

- ACTH stimulation test highlights maximum cortisol values below 18 μg/dL (or < 500 nmol/L) [4].

- Symptomatic hyperandrogenism present in the prepubertal period (early and rapidly evolving pubarche, accelerated bone maturation)—low doses of hydrocortisone (6–10 mg/sqm).

- Alternative treatment options in adolescent and young adult females includes:

- Oral contraceptives containing progestins with low androgenic activity such as desogestrel to induce menstrual cycles and improve acne and hirsutism [4, 7].

- Antiandrogens for patient-important hirsutism that persists despite oral contraceptives [1].

- Eflornithine hydrochloride cream can be used as topical therapy for facial hirsutism. Its effect is of inhibiting the anagen phase of hair production. It is most effective when combined with physical means of hair removal, such as topical lasers [1].

2.7.4 Management of adrenal emergency in CAH

Adrenal crisis is estimated to be responsible for up to 42% of deaths in patients with CAH [1, 5]. Patients with SW are the most exposed to this risk, but not only them. The most common precipitants of this medical emergency are infectious illnesses, gastrointestinal and upper respiratory tract infections, for all ages [1, 5].

Prevention of adrenal crisis is accomplished through patient education on stress dosing (2–3 times usual doses) of glucocorticoid [1, 5]. But there may be situations when oral stress doses will not prevent the progression to adrenal crisis [1]. Each family should have a glucocorticoid injection kit for emergency use at home if oral medication is not tolerated during episodes of major stress [1, 2, 4]. All family members should be trained for its intramuscular administration, especially for patients living far from medical facilities. The injectable dose of hydrocortisone in an emergency is 25 mg for infants, 50 mg for children under 40 kg, and 100 mg for children over 40 kg and for adults [2].

Management of adrenal crisis involves giving an immediate bolus of hydrocortisone 50–100 mg/sqm intravenously or intramuscularly, followed by hydrocortisone 50–100 mg/sqm/day as either continuous infusion or divided at every 6 h [2]. Glucocorticoid doses will be adjusted according to clinical status (state of consciousness, pulse, blood pressure), blood glucose level and serum ionogram. Next day, parenteral administration will be reduced by 1/3 of the dose starting on the day the digestive tolerance reappears and, in parallel with the reduction of parenteral therapy, oral therapy is gradually reintroduced, returning to pre-decompensation doses.

In combination with glucocorticoid therapy, the patient is rehydrated by rapid infusion of intravenous fluids: 1000 mL of 0.9% sodium chloride during the first 60 minutes, or 20 mL/kg up to 60 mL/kg normal saline in children, continuation of therapy will be guided by level of dehydration [1, 2].

If hypoglycemia is present may require dextrose bolus of 0.5–1 g/kg can be given intravenously at 2–3 ml per minute [2].

If the patient has also hyperkalemia, it requires cardiac monitoring for EKG changes and should be treated using insulin with glucose infusion [2].

All patients with CAH should wear medical alert identification tags (Medical Alert bracelet or medallion) indicating the diagnosis of adrenal insufficiency, for prompt therapy initiation in case of emergencies [1, 2, 4].

2.8 Comorbidities asociated with 21OHD

2.8.1 Effect on growth and final adult height

As mentioned earlier, exposure to excessive androgens determines advanced somatic and epiphyseal development accompanied by premature epiphyseal maturation and closure, resulting in a lower final adult height that expected from parental heights. An early diagnosis with the initiation of appropriate treatment could improve the final adult height. However, it is necessary to use an optimal dose of glucocorticoid, avoiding overdose, which could have a negative impact on growth [2, 5].

2.8.2 Impaired bone mineral density (BMD)

Is another consequence of long-term use of supraphysiological doses of glucocorticoid, dexamethasone having the most deleterious effects on BMD compared to hydrocortisone or other intermediate-acting glucocorticoids [1, 5]. In terms of bone metabolism, adrenal androgens including DHEAS can increase BMD, mainly cortical bone [1, 7]. Thus, regarding bone mass late diagnosis and or a poor hormonal control may improve BMD by exposure to higher androgen levels [1]. Similar to the general population, these patients may also benefit from adequate vitamin D intake, a high-calcium diet, and physical activity to prevent bone loss.

2.8.3 Tumor risk

It is estimated that 20–30% of adult patients with CAH have adrenal masses: benign adrenal tumors (29%) or myelolipomas (8.6%). They generally occur in patients with a poor hormonal control, suggesting a role of ACTH stimulation in pathogenesis [5]. There is no evidence that adrenocortical carcinoma is more prevalent in CAH patients [1].

A common and important complication in individuals male with CAH is development of testicular tumors of adrenal-like tissue or testicular adrenal rest tumors (TARTs) [5]. TARTs are bilateral benign testicular tumors, mostly painless, centrally located in the rete testis and easily identified by ultrasound [1, 5]. The central location of TARTs can compress the seminiferous tubules, leading to irreversible damage to the surrounding testicular tissue with gonadal dysfunction and infertility [5]. According to the guidelines, boys with classic CAH should have a testicular ultrasound upon completion of puberty and regular examination for TARTs every 2–5 years [1, 4]. TARTs are rare in NC form, so routine ultrasound is not recommended in NC CAH males [4].

It should be noted that TARTs tumors may also occur in other adrenal enzyme deficiencies like 11β-hydroxylase and 3β-hydroxysteroid dehydrogenase type 2 deficiencies [1].

Due to its strong adrenal-suppressive effect, dexamethasone is preferred in the treatment of TARTs. Testis sparing surgery may be an option, but usually does not improve gonadal function, so this patients may be recommended cryopreservation of sperm before surgery [1].

2.8.4 Fertility

Is affected in both men and women with CAH, especially those with a classic form.

In males fertility is impaired due to hyper- or hypogonadotrophic hypogonadism or through TARTs [2, 7].

In women, elevated androgen and 17OHP levels result in menstrual irregularities and anovulatory cycles [7]. Adverse effects of elevated progesterone on the uterine lining, combined with secondary development of PCOS with oligo-amenorrhea, increases the risk of sub-fertility or infertility [5]. In general, there is an association between the severity of the CAH phenotype and the level of gonadal dysfunction and fertility, mostly reported in women with the salt-wasting subtype [1, 5]. A major cause for low child rates in women with CAH is considered to be a lowest interest in motherhood, especially with the SW phenotype [1]. This may be caused by prenatal androgen exposure that influence gender role behavior, associated with a lack of a partner, dissatisfaction with genital appearance, decreased sexual satisfaction and sexual dysfunction as a result of corrective surgery [1].

2.8.5 Cardiovascular and metabolic disease

Patients with CAH have increased cardiometabolic morbidity [1]. A Swedish population-based study found an increased prevalence of obesity, type 2 diabetes mellitus, obstructive sleep apnoea, hypertension, elevated lipids, atrial fibrillation and venous thromboembolism in CAH individuals compared with control [1, 5]. Regular follow-up with lifestyle interventions to prevent obesity, and screening for diabetes, especially gestational diabetes, and dyslipidemia may improve cardiometabolic outcome [1, 5].

3. 11β-hydroxylase deficiency

CAH owing to 11β-hydroxylase deficiency (11β-OHD) is the second cause of CAH, accounting for 5–8% of all cases [2].

Steroid 11-hydroxylase (CYP11B1, P450c11β) and aldosterone synthase (CYP11B2, P450c11AS, P450aldo) are closely related enzymes, encoded by duplicated genes, and catalyze the final steps in the synthesis of glucocorticoids and mineralocorticoids [1]. CYP11B1 is expressed abundantly in the zona fasciculata, where it converts 11-deoxycortisol to cortisol and deoxycorticosterone (DOC) to corticosterone (**Figure 1**), and also in the zona reticularis, where it initiates the 11-oxo-pathway [1]. CYP11B2 expression is less abundant and confined to the zona glomerulosa where it catalyzes the 11 β-hydroxylase, 18-hydroxylase, and 18-methyloxidase activities which lead to conversion of DOC to aldosterone [1]. This steroid 11-hydroxylase are [1].

11β-OHD occurs as a result of mutations in *CYP11B1*, the gene encoding 11β-hydroxylase, with occurrence of deficient cortisol, and increased DOC and adrenal sex steroids [1]. *CYP11B1* gene is located on the long arm of chromosome 8 (8q24), about 40 kb from the homologous *CYP11B2* gene encoding aldosterone synthase [2]. It consists of 9 exons and 8 introns. Mutations in this gene tend to be grouped into exons 2, 6, 7 and 8. Several types of mutations affecting *CYP11B1* have been described, including missense mutations, splicing, small deletions, small insertions, regulatory deletions, large deletions, or complex rearrangements [9].

The general incidence of this form is estimated to be 1 in 100,000 individuals, and in contrast to 21 hydroxylase deficiency CAH, the disorder is more prevalent in the Middle East and North Africa (1:5000–1:7000 individuals). A mild non-classical form of 11β-OHD CAH has been reported, with an unknown frequency [9].

3.1 Clinical picture

The prominent clinical features of 11β-OHD are female virilization, similar to classical 21OHD and low renin hypertension [9]. Clinically we will encounter virilization in females, childhood gynecomastia, early isosexual/contrasexual pseudopuberty, accelerated bone maturation with reduced adult final height.

Elevated blood pressure is secondary to overproduction of DOC which causes salt retention and hypertension despite the fact that it is a less potent mineralocorticoid than aldosterone [9]. High blood pressure may or may not be associated with hypokalemic metabolic alkalosis and occurs in approximately 2/3 of patients, usually later in childhood or in adolescence [9]. Although the excess of DOC is incriminated, the etiology of hypertension is not fully elucidated. There are other factors involved considering that the decrease in the level of DOC after the administration of dexamethasone is not always associated with BP normalization. Likewise, clinical signs of mineralocorticoid excess and the degree of virilization are not well correlated. Some severely virilized females are normotensive, whereas mildly virilized patients may experience severe hypertension [9].

There have been reported cases of salt loss in neonates with 11β-OHD, incompletely explained pathophysiological, probably due to the natriuretic effect of pregnenolone and progesterone [9]. These episodes could be precipitated by the initiation of glucocorticoid therapy due to a sudden decrease in DOC or by conditions of infectious intercurrences.

Along with the classic form of 11β-OHD there has been described a rare form of non-classical 11β-OH. It presents with excess androgens but without hypertension and has been diagnosed in normotensive children with mild virilization or precocious pubarche and in adults with signs of hyperandrogenemia [9].

3.2 Diagnosis

It is established based on the hormonal profile, that is characterized by:

- Elevated baseline or ACTH-stimulated values of DOC and 11 deoxycortisol

- Elevated urinary metabolites (tetrahydro-11-deoxycortisol, tetrahydro-deoxicorticosterone)

- Moderately elevated 17 OHP levels, that can lead to misdiagnosis of 21OHD at newborn screening [1]

- Elevated androgen levels: androstenedione, testosterone, DHEAS.

4. 3-β hydroxysteroid dehydrogenase deficiency type II

There are 2 human 3β-hydroxysteroid dehydrogenase (HSD3B) genes: type I and type II [1, 9].

HSD3B1 encodes an isozyme found in the placenta, brain, liver, skin. HSD3B2 encodes an isoenzyme found mainly in the adrenals and gonads [1, 9]. Both of these isozymes can convert delta 5 (Δ5) to delta 4 (Δ4) steroids (**Figure 2**) [1, 9]. Mutations in HSD3B2 cause a rare form of CAH, characterized by elevated ratios of Δ5/Δ4 steroids, notably 17OHPreg/17OHP, that are >8 SD above normal [1]. About 45 mutations in HSD3B2 have been described, of which 37 are missense, nonsense, major deletion, or complex rearrangements.

Classical form of HSD3B2 deficiency causes genital ambiguity in both sexes: genetic females are mildly virilized because some fetal adrenal DHEA is converted to testosterone by HSD3B1, that can act on low concentrations of steroids in the circulation; genetic males synthesize some androgens by peripheral conversion of DHEA, but these are insufficient for complete male genital development [1].

Also, hepatic HSD3B1 permits conversion of some of the elevated 17OHPreg to 17OHP, engendering false positives in newborn screening for 21OHD [1].

Diagnosis of HSD3B2 deficiency is based on identification of elevated serum levels of Δ5 steroids and their urinary metabolites (pregnentriol and 16-pregnenetriol) and by elevated ratios of Δ5/Δ4 steroids.

It is worth mentioning that newborns show a physiological increase in steroid levels Δ5. In this case, the diagnosis requires evaluation by the ACTH stimulation

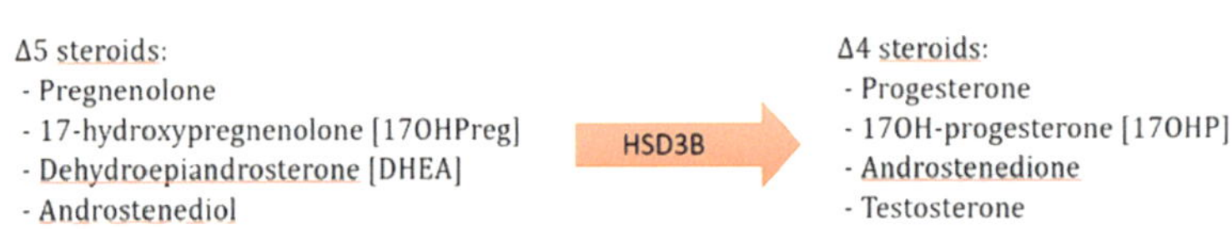
Δ5 steroids:
- Pregnenolone
- 17-hydroxypregnenolone [17OHPreg]
- Dehydroepiandrosterone [DHEA]
- Androstenediol
HSD3B
Δ4 steroids:
- Progesterone
- 17OH-progesterone [17OHP]
- Androstenedione
- Testosterone

Figure 2.
Enzymatic conversion mediated by HSD3B.

test. Increases of more than 2 standard deviations of 17 OH pregnenolone, DHEA, Δ5 17OHPregnenolone/17 OH progesterone ratio and Δ5 17OHPregnenolone/cortisol ratio are considered diagnostic for HSD3B2 deficiency.

Nonclasic form of HSD3B2 deficiency manifest itself in form of precocious development of pubic and axillary hair at both sexes and virilization signs in females.

5. 17α-hydroxylase/17,20 lyase deficiency

17α-hydroxylase (CYP17A1, P450c17) is a double-acting enzyme, both 17α-hydroxylase and 17.20-lyase. The 17α-hydroxylase activity mediate conversion of pregnenolone to 17OHPreg and progesterone to 17OHP, and the 17,20-lyase activity convert 17OH-Preg to DHEA, and to a lesser extent 17OHP to androstenedione [1].

CYP17A1 is absent in zona glomerulosa, has only 17α-hydroxylase activity in zona fasciculata, and is fully expressed, with both activities in the zona reticularis [1].

This enzyme is encoded by the *CYP17A1* gene, located on the long arm of chromosome 10 (10q24.3). Mutations in the CYP17A1 gene with 17-hydroxylase deficiency (17OHD) are rare, account for approximately 1% of all CAH cases, more common in Brazil or China [1, 9]. At least 100 mutations affecting CYP17A1 have been described so far, such as missense/nonsense, splicing, small/large deletions, small insertions, but also complex rearrangements. 17OHD affects steroid synthesis in both the adrenals and gonads [9].

Lack of CYP17A1 blocks sex steroid biosynthesis, thus we will encounter undervirilized genitalia, hypertension, absence of pubertal sexualization and gynecomastia in males, respectively normal aspect of the genitals, hypertension, absence of pubertal sexualization (absence of telarche, primary amenorrhea), minimal body hair in females [1, 9].

Hypertension is caused by overproduction of DOC in the zona fasciculata. 17OHD is accompanied by a lack of cortisol synthesis, with low serum levels of potassium, renine and aldosterone, but very high values of corticosterone substitutes for glucocorticoid requirements [1].

Clinically, the suspicion of 17OHD should be considered in hypertensive patients with hypokalemia and low renin and aldosterone levels, in patients with delayed puberty or stopped developing puberty, in children with karyotype 46, XY with inguinal hernia or female external genitalia. It can also be considered in women with unexplained infertility, who may associate a partial deficit with normal sexualization.

Hormone evaluation will identify elevated values of DOC, corticosterone and 18 OH-corticosterone and gonadotropins, associated with low values of 17 OH pregnenolone and 17 OH-progesterone, renin, and aldosterone [9].

Cases of isolated 17.20 lyase deficiency have been reported [1, 9]. In this situation the conversion of pregnenolone to sex steroid precursors with 19 carbon atoms is blocked, without affecting cortisol synthesis. Clinically we will meet external female genitals at birth, regardless of genetic sex.

6. P450 oxidoreductase deficiency

P450 oxidoreductase (POR) is a flavoprotein that transfers electrons from NADPH to all microsomal cytochrome P450 (CYP) enzymes, including CYP17A1, CYP21A2, CYP19A1 (aromatase, P450aro) [1].

POR mutations will be associated in varying degrees with concomitant decrease in the activity of 17α-hydroxylase/17.20 lyase, 21 α-hydroxylase and aromatase. It is a very rare disease [1]. Splicing, missense, or nonsense mutations, small or large deletions, and small gene insertions affecting the gene located on the long arm of chromosome 7 (7q11.23) cause POR deficiency [9].

Clinical findings are various:

- Possible virilization of the mother associated with low serum estriol levels, which thus becomes a biological marker of disease, highlighted in the triple test performed in the second pregnancy trimester
- Girls with severe degrees of virilization (Prader III or IV)
- Boys with normal external genitalia or sexual infantilism
- During adolescence and adulthood: various degrees of virilization in women, the mildest form being similar to PCOS; various degrees of sub virilization in men, the mildest form presenting only with infertility.

Patients with POR deficiency typically has normal electrolytes and mineralocorticoid function, nearly normal cortisol levels that respond poorly to ACTH stimulation, increased levels of 17OHP, but lower than in the isolated 21OHD, and low levels of sex steroids [1].

7. Congenital lipoid adrenal hyperplasia

To initiate steroidogenesis, cholesterol from cytoplasmic storage depots is transported to the inner mitochondrial membrane by steroidogenic acute regulatory protein (StAR), a transporter protein. At this level CYP11A1 (P450scc) will converted it to pregnenolone [1].

Mutations in StAR cause a rare form of CAH called congenital lipoid adrenal hyperplasia. In this disorder we have hormone deficiency on all 3 lines: mineralocorticoid, glucocorticoid, and sex steroids. Furthermore, lipoid CAH is typically associated with very large adrenals secondary to the accumulation of cholesterol esters in the adrenal glands [1].

From a clinical point of view, children have normal length and weight at birth; male newborns have a completely female phenotype but lack the mullerian derivatives; adrenal insufficiency is manifest from birth, with severe salt loss and dehydration; in 2/3 of cases, we find skin hyperpigmentation and in 1/4 cases hypoglycemia during infancy [9].

Attenuated forms are also described, in which the salt loss becomes manifest later, after the age of 1 month. Female patients with a minor deficiency may have a normal phenotype in childhood, but with the absence of puberty or spontaneous puberty, but stopped in evolution.

These patients will have electrolyte imbalances with severe hyponatremia and hyperkalemia, very low levels of cortisol, aldosterone, DHEA, but also their precursors with much higher levels of ACTH, plasma renin and gonadotropins, the latter even in middle childhood.

The treatment of this condition is common with the classic forms of CAH with adequate glucocorticoid and mineralocorticoid substitution.

8. Conclusions

Under the name of congenital adrenal hyperplasia, there is a heterogeneous spectrum of diseases whose phenotype depends on the type and degree of enzyme deficiency. The diagnosis has an important impact on both the patient and his family. Given that 21 hydroxylase deficiency is the most common etiopathogenesis of the disease, it often becomes synonymous with congenital adrenal hyperplasia. However, we must also consider the possibility of the existence of other enzymatic defects. In conclusion, we are talking about a group of complex diseases whose diagnosis and management require a multidisciplinary approach with the formation of a team of experts in neonatology, endocrinology, genetics, surgery, psychology, these patients requiring regular long-term evaluation.

Acknowledgements

The authors would like to thank to their teachers, professor doctor Constantin Dumitrache and professor doctor Mihail Coculescu, from which they inherited the passion for the secrets of endocrinology.

Conflict of interest

The authors declare no conflict of interest.

Author details

Adina Mariana Ghemigian* and Nicoleta Dumitru
C.I. Parhon National Institute of Endocrinology, “Carol Davila” University of Medicine and Pharmacy, Bucharest, Romania

*Address all correspondence to: adinaghemi@yahoo.com

References

[1] Claahsen-van der Grinten HL, Speiser PW, Ahmed SF, Arlt W, Auchus RJ, Falhammar H, et al. Congenital adrenal hyperplasia-current insights in pathophysiology, diagnostics, and management. Endocrine Reviews. 2022;**43**(1):91-159. DOI: 10.1210/endrev/bnab016

[2] Yau M, Gujral J, New MI. Congenital adrenal hyperplasia: Diagnosis and emergency treatment. 2019 Apr 16. In: Feingold KR, Anawalt B, Boyce A, Chrousos G, de Herder WW, Dhatariya K, et al., editors. Endotext [Internet]. South Dartmouth (MA): MDText.com, Inc.; 2000 [Accessed: May 16, 2022]

[3] Arriba M, Ezquieta B. Molecular diagnosis of steroid 21-hydroxylase deficiency: A practical approach. Frontiers in Endocrinology. 2022;**29**(13):834549. DOI: 10.3389/fendo.2022.834549

[4] Speiser PW, Arlt W, Auchus RJ, Baskin LS, Conway GS, Merke DP, et al. Congenital adrenal hyperplasia due to steroid 21-hydroxylase deficiency: An endocrine society clinical practice guideline. Journal of Endocrinology and Metabolism. 2018;**103**(11):4043-4088. DOI: 10.1210/jc.2018-01865. [Erratum in: The Journal of Clinical Endocrinology and Metabolism 2019;**104**(1):39-40]

[5] Mallappa A, Merke DP. Management challenges and therapeutic advances in congenital adrenal hyperplasia. Nature Reviews Endocrinology. 2022;**18**(6): 337-352. DOI: 10.1038/s41574-022-00655-w. Epub 2022 Apr 11

[6] Nimkarn S, Gangishetti PK, Yau M, et al. 21-Hydroxylase-deficient congenital adrenal hyperplasia. 2002 Feb 26 [Updated 2016 Feb 4]. In: Adam MP, Mirzaa GM, Pagon RA, et al., editors. GeneReviews® [Internet]. Seattle (WA): University of Washington, Seattle; 1993-2022. Available from: https://www.ncbi.nlm.nih.gov/books/NBK1171/. [Accessed: June 02, 2022]

[7] Nordenström A, Falhammar H. Management of endocrine disease: Diagnosis and management of the patient with non-classic CAH due to 21-hydroxylase deficiency. European Journal of Endocrinology. 2019;**180**(3):R127-R145. DOI: 10.1530/EJE-18-0712

[8] van der Kamp HJ, Wit JM. Neonatal screening for congenital adrenal hyperplasia. European Journal of Endocrinology. 2004;**151**(Suppl. 3): U71-U75. DOI: 10.1530/eje.0.151u071

[9] New M, Yau M, Lekarev O, et al. Congenital adrenal hyperplasia. [Updated 2017 Mar 15]. In: Feingold KR, Anawalt B, Boyce A, et al., editors. Endotext [Internet]. South Dartmouth (MA): MDText.com, Inc.; 2000. Available from: https://www.ncbi.nlm.nih.gov/books/NBK278953/. [Accessed: June 03, 2022]

Chapter 6

Congenital Adrenal Hyperplasia – The Main Effect of 21-Hydroxylase Deficiency

Berta Carvalho, Filipa Carvalho and Davide Carvalho

Abstract

Congenital adrenal hyperplasia (CAH) consists of a group of autosomal recessive disorders resulting from enzymatic defects in steroidogenesis. More than 95% of CAH cases result from a deficiency of the 21-hydroxylase enzyme, which leads to cortisol deficiency, with or without aldosterone insufficiency, and also an excess of androgen. The clinical spectrum varies from milder symptoms to severe cases settled by the functional impairment of the corresponding pathogenic variant in the *CYP21A2* gene. The two major forms of CAH caused by 21-hydroxylase deficiency are the classical form and the non-classic, or late onset form. There are two subtypes of the classic form: salt wasting and simple virilized. Diagnosis is clinically confirmed by 17OH-progesterone measurements, although genotyping is now progressively assuming an essential role for characterising patients. Genotyping is sometimes challenging, due to the existence of the highly homologous *CYP21A1P* pseudogene. The 21-hydroxylase enzyme is encoded by the *CYP21A2* gene, where most of the pathogenic variants defects are due to meiotic recombination phenomena events between the *CYP21A2* and *CYP21A1P*. Complete gene analysis is recommended to obtain a correct diagnosis and a better understanding of the underlying mechanisms of the disease in patients with CAH, and is relevant for prognosis and for prescribing the appropriate type of genetic counselling.

Keywords: CAH, cortisol, aldosterone, androgens, 21-hydroxylase, *CYP21A2*

1. Introduction

Congenital adrenal hyperplasia (CAH) consists of a group of autosomal recessive disorders caused by a defective activity of one of the enzymes involved in the steroidogenic pathway on the zona fasciculata of adrenal cortex, leading to an impairment in cortisol synthesis by the adrenal gland [1–5]. From the several enzymes involved in the adrenal steroids pathway, the 21-hydroxylase (21-OH) enzyme is responsible for the majority of CAH cases [5, 6]. Less frequently, other rare deficits in other enzymes may occur, namely: 11β-hydroxylase (11β-OH), 17α-hydroxylase (17α-OH), 3β-hydroxisteroid dehydrogenase (3β-HSD), and StaR protein cholesterol side chain and cholesterol 20–22-desmolase. 21-OH, which is an enzyme belonging to

IntechOpen

the cytochrome P450 enzyme group, is responsible for the conversion of progesterone into deoxycorticosterone and for the conversion of 17-hydroxyprogesterone (17-OHP) into 11-deoxycortisol [7, 8]. The impairment of this enzyme leads to the accumulation of precursor substrates for 21-hydroxylation, particularly 17-hydroxyprogesterone (17-OHP), which in turn causes elevated levels of androstenedione, testosterone, dihydrotestosterone, and other peripherally estrogens [4, 7–9]. Deficits in cortisol or aldosterone and the consequent excess of androgens caused by the accumulation of precursors may be responsible for distinct levels of enzyme activity, leading to different forms of the disease, ranging from severe, moderate, to mild. This monogenic autosomal disorder is transmitted in a recessive pattern, requiring two mutated alleles for the disease to occur [8]. The clinical manifestations are distinct and, in general, correspond to the enzymatic activity of the less-affected allele [6, 10, 11]. Approximately 95% of CAH cases are the result of an impairment of the 21-hydroxylase enzyme, which is one of the several enzymes involved in the androgens pathway. Pathogenic variants of the encoding *CYP21A2* gene may lead to a partial or complete loss of function and an impairment of cortisol and aldosterone synthesis. In turn, the depletion of cortisol concentration may inhibit the negative feedback loop, leading to a compensatory release of the corticotrophin release hormone (CRH) and the adrenocorticotropic hormone (ACTH) by the hypothalamus and the pituitary gland, respectively, and also an adrenal cortex hyperplasia.

The phenotypic spectrum of CAH is widely variable, and the major clinical manifestations of adrenal insufficiency caused by aldosterone and cortisol deficits and androgen excess constitute the main clinical concern, with morbidity and mortality becoming less common. Therapy with hormone replacement constitutes a considerable benefit for patients since early diagnosis, although precise and individualised treatment is required for better outcomes.

Genetic counselling is essential, especially because this disease affects many individuals of reproductive age [1–3], and for the elucidation of the consequences and complications for offspring. Molecular analysis of the gene responsible for 21-OH deficiency is a necessary tool for the confirmation of clinical diagnosis of the affected individual, which can also provide added valuable information for relatives or offspring at risk.

2. Clinical manifestations of CAH due to 21-OH deficiency

Based on distinct phenotypes, the disease was classified into two forms: the classic form, subdivided into the salt-wasting (SW) and simple virilising (SV) forms, and the non-classical or late-onset form (**Table 1**) [12]. In both forms, decreased cortisol synthesis causes increased secretion of ACTH, which in turn stimulates the adrenal gland to produce cortisol precursors, including androgens and their intermediates (DHEAS, androstenedione and testosterone). In this way, hyperplasia of the adrenal cortex is caused, as mentioned above [13].

2.1 Salt-wasting (SW) form

The SW form of CAH is the most severe form of this disease, accounting for 75% of cases of the classic form of the disease [13]. This form is characterised by a complete absence of enzymatic activity, with consequent cortisol and aldosterone deficiency [14]. SW form patients present alterations in the body electrolyte balance

	Classic		Non- classic
	Salt Wasting	**Simple Virilizing**	
Age at diagnosis	NB till 6 months	Fem: NB till 2y; Male; 2 to 4y	Infancy till young adulthood
Genitalia	Fem: ambiguous Male: normal	Fem: ambiguous Male: normal	Fem: virilized Male: normal
Incidence	1:20000	1: 60000	1: 10000
Hormones			
Aldosterone	↓	N	N
Renin (PRA)	↑	N or ↑	N
Cortisol	↓	↓	N
18 OHP	> 50 ng/mL	25 to 50 ng/mL	5 to 25 ng/mL (after ACTH stimulation test)
Testosterone	↑	↑	Variable to ↑
Growth	-2 to -3SD	-1 to −2 SD	Probably N
21-hydroxylase activity (%)	0	<1–2	20 to 60
Typical pathogenic variants (*CYP21A2*)	Gene deletions and large conversions – 8 bp del; E6 cluster; p.Gln319Ter (Q318X); p.Arg357Trp (R356W)	p.Ile173Asn (I172N)	p.Pro31Leu (P30L); p.Val282Leu (V281L); p.Pro454Ser (P453S)

NB - Newborn; Fem – Female; PRA - Plasma Renin Activity.

Table 1.
Clinical characteristics, hormonal levels and genotype–phenotype correlation for the most common pathogenic variants, according to the percentage of enzyme activity.

due to the deficient production of mineralocorticoids. Appropriate therapy should be administered in a timely manner, as this form can range from severe forms to more discrete cases, with increased plasma renin activity [15]. In all cases, the decreased production of cortisol and aldosterone poses a threat to survival, with acute adrenal insufficiency occurring between the 1st and 3rd weeks of life [16]. Approximately 50% of salt wasting crisis occur between the age of 6 to 14 years old [15]. In the SV forms, external genitalia may also be affected, caused by a deficiency in cortisol and the consequent increase in adrenal androgens [9]. Affected males typically presented severe electrolyte imbalances within the first 2 weeks of life, however, in general, they do not show signs of excess androgen production, with only hyperpigmentation of the genital area occurring (**Table 1**) [17]. The excess of androgens produced during pregnancy in individuals with 21-OH cause the virilization of female foetuses, resulting in pseudohermaphroditism [4]. Prior to the onset of newborn screening programmess, affected females were more rapidly identified, on account of the simultaneous presence of genital ambiguity.

2.2 Simple Virilizing (SV) form

In the SV form of CAH there is a partial enzymatic deficit, which is manifested by a decrease in cortisol [18]. SV CAH patients present hypocortisolism and simple

Classic Salt-Wasting—severe form
(0% enzymatic activity)
Failure to thrive
Cortisol deficiency
Mineralocorticoid deficiency
Hyponatremia
Hyperkalemia
High Plasma Renin Activity (or renin)
Hypovolemic shock
Excess androgen production, early in life
Virilization of external genitalia in females
Classic Simple Virilizing—intermediate severity form
(1–2% enzymatic activity)
Virilization of external genitalia in females
Progressive premature pubarche
Progressive virilization with clitoromegaly (female) or increased penile size (male)
Elevated androgen levels cause accelerated growth velocity and advanced bone age but premature fusion of the epiphyses is also observed causing final short stature.
Non-Classic Adrenal Hyperplasia—mild form
(20–50% enzymatic activity)
Between asymptomatic or with signs of androgen excess appearing later in life (acne; hirsutism; menstrual irregularities; anovulation; infertility)

Table 2.
Phenotypes of 21-hydroxylase deficiency.

virilisation. Furthermore, in the perinatal period, newborn female foetuses may present ambiguous genitalia without overt salt loss in affected females (**Table 2**) [19]. Virilization can be classified according to the Prader Stages scale, which ranges from 1 to 5, with Stage 5 being the most severe. Despite these external features, the female internal organs are not affected [4]. Male children may also present signs of early virilization, due to excess androgens, however, the undervaluation of signs of early virilization can delay the diagnosis of this disease in male individuals [4, 16].

2.3 Non-classical (NC) form

In the NC form of CAH due to 21-OH deficiency, the enzymatic impairment is partial and usually there is no cortisol deficiency [20]. This form is less severe and of late onset and manifests itself by signs of precocious puberty and gynaecological anomalies, which may occur either in late childhood or in early adulthood [14] (**Table 2**). Some affected women have no symptoms at all, and a considerable high number of men remain asymptomatic and only have a genetic diagnosis during segregation family analysis [20].

3. Prevalence in different ethnic populations

The overall incidence of classical CAH due 21-OH deficiency is 1:10,000–15,000 births, with a carriers' frequency of approximately 1:60–100 [3, 4, 10, 21]. Heterozygosity for 21-OH deficiency in the classical form is estimated to be 1:60 in non-Jewish Caucasians and 1:3 in Ashkenazy Jews [7, 8, 22]. The incidence is much lower in Afro-Americans, ranging from 1:25,000 to 1:42,000 in different studies [10, 11]. The most common form of CAH is the NC form, or the late onset form, which affects between 0.1% and 1% of the overall population. The NC-CAH form presents non-specific features, oligomenorrhea, hirsutism and infertility, which causes an ascertainment bias which in turn leads to a diagnosis of a higher number of affected females. Affected males are mostly identified during family screening studies, since androgen excess manifestations are not commonly recognised. NC-CAH patients do not often oversecrete CRH and ACTH, although some patients might demonstrate an increase in glucocorticoids response to ACTH stimulation, reflecting a subtle adrenal hyperplasia [9, 14]. The increase of the secretion of androgens by adrenal glands without an overstimulation of ACTH can be justified by the alteration in kinetic enzymatic activity of CYP21A2 [22]. In addition, an increased level of androgens in NC-CAH may be the result of the peripheral conversion of precursors, or can be due to ovarian hypersecretion, as NC-CAH women frequently have polycystic ovaries.

Among hirsute women, the prevalence of CAH attains between 1% and 10% [17, 22, 23]. A clinical study based on ACTH-stimulated 17-OHP concentrations reported the incidence to be highest among Ashkenazi Jewish populations [24]. In addition, Ashkenazi Jews are reported to have the pathogenic variant p.Val282Leu with a high allelic frequency of approximately 63%, which is mostly associated with non-classic CAH. On the contrary, p.Val282Leu was not detected in Yupik-speaking, Eskimos of Western Alaska, Native Americans, East Indians and Asians. Interestingly, the Yupik Eskimos, represent an isolated geographic population and the splice site intronic variation c.293-13A/C > G in intron 2 is found to be represent a founder effect for this population [25].

Several studies regarding the genotyping of 21-OH deficiency have been presented over recent years. A large study conducted on the French CAH population showed a frequency of the most common pathogenic variants, for the classic form, of 30% of c.293-13A/C > G in intron 2, 25% for large rearrangements, 17% for p.Ile173Asn (I172N) in exon 4, and 7% of p.Gln319* (Q318X) in exon 8. For the NC form, the same study found a frequency of 55% for p.Val282Leu (V281L), 9% for c.293-13A/C > G, 8% for large rearrangements, 4% for p.Ile173Asn, and 3% for p.Gln319* [25]. In Brazil, three novel pathogenic variants were described, namely: an insertion of adenine 1003∧1004 insA in exon 4, a transition C > T in codon 408 (p.Arg408Cys), and a transition A > G in intron 2, IVS2 – 2A > G, which it is suggested is due a founder effect, as it had previously been found in the G424S pathogenic variant in the same population [26–28].

In Finland, multiple pathogenic variants have been analysed and found to have an independent founder effect, with each one being associated with a distinct haplotype, where some are identical to other European populations. This is probably due to remote immigration phenomena originating from the Scandinavian or the Baltic countries, as well as other specificities from that population, albeit with a more recent origin.

In Tunisia, the pathogenic variant p.Gln319* (Q318X) was found to be the most prevalent in that population (35.8%) [29].

A study of the population of Iran showed the contrary, demonstrating that the common deletion of 8 nt in exon 3 is the most frequent pathogenic variant of the *CYP21A2* gene (10%), followed by the c.293-13A/C > G, p.Ile173Asn, and the promotor deletion in the gene. Unlike other populations, p.Arg357Trp (R356W) in exon 8, was not found in Iran [30].

Gene rearrangements, such as the large 3 kb deletion, are frequent among the Anglo-Saxon population (28%). Furthermore, the frameshift pathogenic variant p.Gln319* in exon 8 of *CYP21A2* gene was found in 16% of East Indians and among Croatians, the missense p.Arg356Trp variant is one of the most frequent pathogenic variants (14%) [29].

The pathogenic variant in exon 7, p.Val282Leu is often found in NC-CAH forms and represented 86% of all alleles studied [31, 32]. *De novo* rearrangements and deletions/conversions of *CYP21A2* gene represent 1% of the affected alleles. Several forms of the chimeric *CYP21A2/CYP21A1P* gene have been described in different populations [33, 34].

4. Differential diagnosis

4.1 Biochemical

The biochemical diagnosis of CAH is made using hormone assays. 17-hydroxyprogesterone (17-OHP) is the gold standard screening marker for this disease [16], however other markers can also be used, such as DHEA, cortisol, testosterone, aldosterone, and renin (or plasma renin activity). Individuals with the classic form of CAH present a marked increase in serum 17-OHP, with values greater than 100 ng/mL, without an increase in 11-deoxycortisol and with a less marked increase in basal dehydroepiandrosterone and testosterone [14]. In patients presenting a SW form, there is also an increase in plasma renin activity, and manifestations such as hyponatremia and hyperkalemia [19]. CAH carriers frequently present normal basal 17-OHP levels and diagnostic strategy involves stimulation with synthetic ACTH with subsequent hormone measurement after 60 minutes. A concentration of 17-OHP greater than 15 ng/mL is indicative of an impairment in 21-OH activity, however many carriers' individuals have only slightly increase hormone concentration after stimulation [7].

4.2 Molecular genetics

Molecular genetic testing of the *CYP21A2* gene is considered to be essential for the establishment of correlations between genotype and phenotype, as well as the confirmation of clinical and biochemical diagnosis, measuring the status of severity of the patients, distinguishing between severe and milder cases, and, very importantly, making the decision regarding the appropriate genetic counselling for at risk family members and their couples. The molecular diagnosis of CAH is based on the identification of point pathogenic variants and small deletions or insertions, which are mostly transferred from the pseudogene to the active gene [35]. The molecular analysis of the *CYP21A2* gene involves amplification with specific primers just for the *CYP21A2* gene, in order to ensure the targeting of the functional gene, instead of the inactive pseudogene [12, 36]. As *CYP21A2* is constituted by 10 exons and intronic regions of reduced size, it is possible to amplify the entire gene, enabling the possibility to analyse all exons and their intron-exon flanking regions. The most common strategy employed to achieve this specificity is to select a primer that is located at the site with a specific and unique gene sequence [8]. The presence of sequence variations can cause alterations in the sequence reading and interpretation and different forward or reverse primers have to be used to achieve a complete analysis, emphasising the complexity of CAH genomics.

4.2.1 Structure of the CYP21A2 gene

21-OH CAH deficiency is mainly caused by pathogenic variants in the *CYP21A2* gene, which is the gene that encodes the 21-OH enzyme [21]. *CYP21A2* is located in the Major Histocompatibility Complex (MHC) class III region, on the short arm of chromosome 6 (6p21.3), which is a region that displays a complex organisation of genes with high variability in gene size and copy numbers [37, 38] (**Figure 1**). Approximately 30 kb apart from the *CYP21A2* gene is a pseudogene – *CYP21A1P*. Both the *CYP21A2* gene and the *CYP21A1P* pseudogene share 98% homology between exons and 96% in introns, and both are constituted by 10 exons, spanning 3.1 kb [21, 39, 40].

Throughout evolution, the inactive *CYP21A1P* pseudogene has acquired multiple pathogenic variants, as well as small insertions or deletions and point pathogenic variants that prevent the synthesis of a normal functional protein. The high degree of homology between the gene and the pseudogene enables the occurrence of unequal pairing during meiosis between homologous chromosomes and sister chromatids [41]. Approximately 95% of pathogenic variants in the *CYP21A2* gene result from meiotic recombination events between the gene and the pseudogene [8], with approximately 75% of pathogenic variants resulting from conversion events of large sequences from the pseudogene to the gene or punctual conversion of single alterations (microconversion). Approximately 20% of the pathogenic variants found in this gene are the result of an unequal crossing-over during meiosis, leading to the occurrence of duplications and/or deletions. Large gene conversions and deletions may result in the *CYP21A1P/CYP21A2* chimeric genes, comprising around 20% of the pathogenic variants. The remaining 5% correspond to new pathogenic variants which are not related with recombination events and *de novo* pathogenic variants account for approximately 1–2% of cases [41]. Three other genes are placed adjacent and alternately to *CYP21A2* and *CYP21A1P*, namely the *RP1*, *C4*, *TNXB* genes, as well as two pseudogene – *RP2* and *TNXA* [42]. This configuration is designated by the RCCX module (RP-C4-CYP21-TNX) and it extends to approximately 30 kb, where the orientation from telomere to centromere is: *RP1-C4A-CYP21A1P-TNXA-RP2-C4B-CYP21A2-TNXB* (**Figure 1**) [42]. The *C4B* and *C4A* genes encode for the fourth component of serum complement [41] and the *TNXB* gene encodes for an extracellular matrix protein termed tenascin-X23. In turn, *RP1* encodes a DNA helicase nuclear protein [42]. The RCCX module organisation is usually bimodular, one with the active *CYP21A2* gene, and the other with the inactive pseudogene *CYP21A1P*, which is present in around 69% of the Caucasian population. Monomodular presentation is present in around 17% of the population, whereas trimodular haplotype occurs in almost 14% of cases [33, 42].

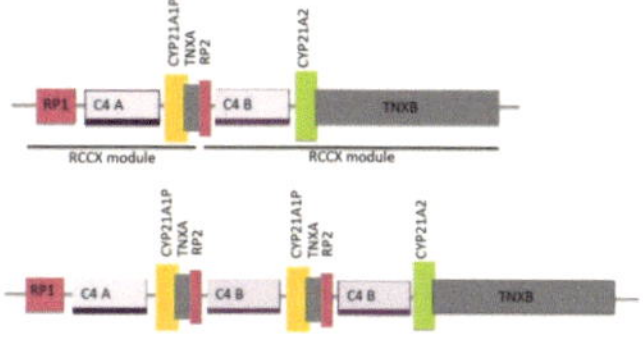

Figure 1.
RCCX modules: Bimodular haplotype (upper) and a three modular haplotype with two modules harbouring the CYP21A1P pseudogene and one the CYP21A2 gene.

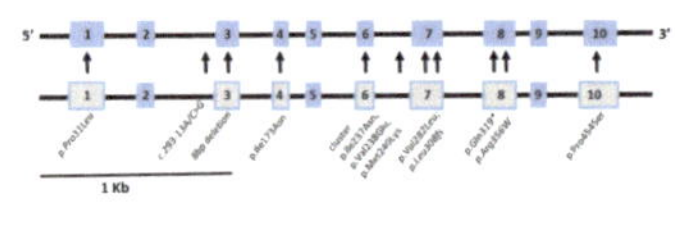

Figure 2.
CYP21A2 and CYP21A1P interconversion events responsible for the conversion of the most common pathogenic variants from the pseudogene to CYP21A2 gene.

The monomodular organisation is characterised by a deletion of 26 or 32 kb, depending on whether the *C4B* is a short or a long gene, without or with the HERV-K sequence. Several deletions have been described, giving rise to different chimera *CYP21A1P*/*CYP21A2* genes [34]. The most common deletion involves the 3′ end of *CYP21A1P*, the entire *C4B* gene, and the 5′ end of the *CYP21A2* gene, which produces a single non-functional chimeric gene with 5′ and 3′ ends of *CYP21A1P* and *CYP21A2*, respectively (**Figure 2**).

The trimodular haplotype may exhibit two copies of the *CYP21A1P* gene and one copy of the *CYP21A2* gene, or two copies of the *CYP21A2* gene and one copy of the *CYP21A1P* pseudogene, the latter being described in patients who present both the p.Gln319* pathogenic variant and chimeric *CYP21A1P*/*CYP21A2* genes together [35, 36, 43]. The existence of different haplotype with simultaneous distinct copy number variation with a large number of sequence variants presents a challenge for the characterisation of *CYP21A2* alleles. Pathogenic variants have been described along the entire gene, in the coding region, as well as in the intron-exon boundaries and beyond, and also in the 5′ and 3′ untranslated region, which demands a careful full gene analysis.

CAH can also be caused by uniparental isodisomy events, although this phenomenon is less frequent [44]. To date, more than 1000 genetic variants have been reported, but only a quarter of them affect human health, with most of these resulting in classic CAH cases [45]. Several sequence variants have been described in the non-translated regions of the gene and even in the promoter sequence, many of them associated with NC-CAH [46]. 153 of the 230 genetic variants were demonstrated to be missense pathogenic variants [45] and these can result in all forms of the disease, whereas nonsense and frameshift pathogenic variants are prone to result in classical forms.

4.2.2 CYP21A2 gene pathogenic variants

The use of the screening approach for the detection of the ten most common pathogenic variants was the most-used practice among molecular genetic laboratories for several years, providing a molecular confirmation for the majority of cases. The most common pathogenic variants evaluated in classic and non-classic forms were responsible for almost 80% of the cases of CAH caused by 21-OH deficiency:

- **p.Pro31Leu (P30L or Pro30Leu):** This pathogenic variant has an enzyme activity of around 20–60% in cultured cells [45], however this enzyme activity is quickly lost when cells are lysed, pointing to a relative instability of this enzyme. p.Pro31Leu is associated with the mild form of disease and is found in one sixth of NC-alleles, although it can be present with a higher prevalence in specific ethnicities, such as the Japanese [47]. NC-CAH patients who carry this pathogenic variant may present more serious manifestations of androgen excess than those patients who carry the most common pathogenic variants associated with NC forms, with p.Val282Leu being associated as having a dominant effect on patients [48].

- **p.Pro31Leu (P30L or Pro30Leu):** This pathogenic variant has an enzyme activity of around 20–60% in cultured cells [45], however this enzyme activity is quickly lost when cells are lysed, pointing to a relative instability of this enzyme. p.Pro31Leu is associated with the mild form of disease and is found in one sixth of NC-alleles, although it can be present with a higher prevalence in specific ethnicities, such as the Japanese [47]. NC-CAH patients who carry this pathogenic variant may present more serious manifestations of androgen excess than those patients who carry the most common pathogenic variants associated with NC forms, with p.Val282Leu being associated as having a dominant effect on patients [48].

- **c.293-13A/C > G (IVS2–13A/C > G: A or C-G Pathogenic Variant in Intron 2):** This pathogenic variant is defined by a substitution of an adenine or cytosine nucleotide to a guanine, at 13 bp before the end of intron 2. This alteration is responsible for the alternative splicing of intron 2, which is characterised by a retention of 19 nucleotides, as well as usually the disruption of mRNA and a shift in the translation reading frame with a generation of a premature stop codon [49].

- **p.Gly111Valfs∗21 (Del 8 bp or G11018nt):** This pathogenic variant is characterised by a deletion of 8 nucleotide in exon 3, resulting in a frameshift variant with nil enzyme activity. Although this pathogenic variant is mainly associated with SW forms of CAH [50, 51].

- **p.Ile173Asn (I172N or Ile172Asn):** This pathogenic variant is marked by a nucleotide missense substitution that causes the shift of isoleucine by asparagine aminoacid. This alteration is associated with approximately 1% of normal activity and is mainly found in the SV forms of CAH, although it has also been described as being present in SW forms of CAH [51].

- **p.Ile237Asn, p.Val238Glu, p.Met239Lys (Cluster in Exon 6: I236N/V237E/M238K or Ile-Val-Met236–237-238-Asn-Glu-Lys):** The cluster of three missense pathogenic variants in the G helix supresses enzymatic activity, probably through interference with substrate binding [49].

- **p.Val282Leu (V281L or Val281Leu):** The p.Val282Leu occurs in the majority of patients with NC 21-hydroxylase deficiency form who carry the HLA haplotype B14; DR1, this association being consistent with a founder effect [52]. Overall, approximately 70% of all NC alleles carry the p.Val282Leu pathogenic variant [53]. This pathogenic variant results in an enzyme with 40–60% of normal activity when 17-OHP is the substrate, but with only 20% of normal activity for progesterone [54, 55].

- **p.Leu307PhefsTer5 (F306 + T or L306insT):** This nonsense pathogenic variant occurs due to an insertion of 1 thymine nucleotide in exon 7. This variant is often described as a conversion of exons 7 and 8 derived from pseudogene, particularly in the cases of Dutch patients [54].

- **p.Gln319* (Q318X or Gln318-Term):** This pathogenic variant is caused by a nucleotide substitution that shifts the CAG codon to a TAG codon, resulting in a premature stop of protein translation which in turn leads to a non-functional protein [56].

- **p.Arg357Trp (R356W or Arg356Trp):** This missense pathogenic variant is mostly associated with classic CAH forms and the enzyme activity is nil. This alteration is located in exon 8, in a region encoding the K helix of the enzyme, suggesting that interaction with cytochrome P450 reductase (POR) may be affected, although experimental studies are lacking [55].

- **p.Pro454Ser (P453S or Pro453Ser):** This missense pathogenic variant in exon 10 of the gene was initially described as being absent in the pseudogene and is associated with a 50–68% decrease of enzyme activity [57]. It occurs differently in several populations, which suggests that *CYP21A1P* may carry p.Pro454Ser as an occasional polymorphism and that this pathogenic variant is transferred to *CYP21A2* in the same way as the other pathogenic variants frequently cause 21-hydroxylase deficiency [32].

Many other different pathogenic variants have been described, some of which are from wide families, while many others are private from particular families. Most of the pathogenic variants associated with CAH due to 21-OH deficiency are missense pathogenic variants. Their study requires functional studies to be correlated with a clinical form, although nonsense, frameshift, and rearrangement pathogenic variants are promptly deduced as being severe. Genotype–phenotype correlation data demonstrated that some variants were associated with the severe SW form, some with the SV form, and others with the NC form. It was also observed that some of these pathogenic variants confer different phenotypes, depending on whether they are isolated or are associated with another pathogenic variant, resulting in a synergistic effect [57]. Some sequence variants do not affect the protein production and are considered to be benign variants [57]. Some of these sequence variants are also present in *CYP21A1P* gene and can also be transferred by conversion events, although they do not affect the enzyme activity and have no effect on the clinical phenotype.

4.2.3 Targeted screening of the ten most common pathogenic variants

For several years, the study of *CYP21A2* gene was based on the evaluation of the ten most frequent pathogenic variants. Several different molecular methods and strategies have been described to cover just a limited number of pathogenic variants. Polymerase chain reaction (PCR), specific primer sequence (SSCP), restriction fragment length polymorphism (RFLP), and direct DNA Sanger sequencing were among the methods available for screening. The initial screening for the most frequent pathogenic variants included the search for large deletions or conversions events involving the promoter region of the *CYP21A2* gene (del/conv of promoter region), as well as pointing to the following pathogenic variants along the *CYP21A2* gene: exon 1, p.Pro31Leu; intron 2, which is a splicing pathogenic variant c.293–13A/C > G; exon 3, which is a 8 bp deletion (p.Gly111Valfs21); exon 4, p.Ile173Asn; exon 6, which is a cluster of three point pathogenic variants (p.Ile237Asn, p.Val238Glu, p.Met240Lys); exon 7, p.Val282Leu, and a thymine insertion (p.Leu307PhefsX5); exon 8, p.Gln319*, and p.Arg357Trp; and p.Pro454Ser in exon 10 [8].

The study of the large deletions/conversions involving the promoter region of the *CYP21A2* gene was achieved by a PCR-based experiment, followed by digestion with the *Taq I* restriction enzyme [8]. This method covers a large number of pathogenic variants found in CAH patients who are affected by 21-OH deficiency owing to alterations in *CYP21A2*, as the screening strategy fails to identify other pathogenic variants outside the target regions.

4.2.4 Complete gene analysis by sanger sequencing

Whole gene sequencing is nowadays the gold standard for genotyping the *CYP21A2* gene. The full gene analysis of *CYP21A2* by Sanger sequencing allows the detection of the above-described pathogenic variants, as well as the identification of new sequence variations. Specific gene amplification by PCR has dramatically improved the sensitivity of the various techniques available to detect *CYP21A2* pathogenic variants. However, the existence of a highly homologous *CYP21A1P* pseudogene which carries most of the pathogenic variants of interest has revealed the major difficulty in finding a strategy for the selective amplification of the *CYP21A2* gene, owing to the lack of specific primers. Indeed, locus-specific mutation primers and PCR conditions were revised and now enable the gene-specific amplification of *CYP21A2*. Gene sequencing usually analyses both the coding regions and the flanking intron-exon regions of the gene. *CYP21A2* whole genomic sequence may be performed by selecting the *CYP21A2* functional gene and amplification by PCR into two partially-overlapping fragments, with 1517 and 2214 base-pairs (bp), avoiding the co-amplification of the pseudogene *CYP21A1P* [58]. After the selective amplification of the targeted genes and their subsequent purification, the PCR products are sequenced with internal primers that cover the entire *CYP21A2* gene [59].

4.2.5 Large rearrangements

The molecular approach for the identification of large rearrangements is distinct from that used for the analysis of sequence pathogenic variants.

A diversity of methods is available for the detection of large rearrangements in the exonic and/or intronic regions of *CYP21A2* gene and also in the promoter and contiguous regions, such as for neighbours' genes (e.g., *C4B* gene). The southern blot technique has been used as a gold standard for many years in the study of large deletions in the *CYP21A2* gene, however this technique has now been substituted by MLPA (Multiplex Ligation-dependent Probe Amplification). The MLPA experimental technique enables the detection of large rearrangements, where several gene sequences can be simultaneously analysed. The detection of known deletions and duplications in the *CYP21A2* gene and in the *CYP21A1P* pseudogene is currently achieved by using this method, which analyses the variations in the copy number of several exons of the gene, and also identifies sequence variations, as well as contiguous genes and control sequences.

This semi-quantitative method is a simple, reliable, and highly sensitive approach for detecting copy number variations in genomic sequences based on the hybridisation of probes to locus-specific targets and the amplification of the effectively-matched targets. The products of amplification are then separated by capillary electrophoresis and comparison is made between a peak-area pattern obtained from reference and the tested samples enable the determination of which probes/locus have aberrant copy numbers [60, 61].

Another eligible method for detecting copy number variations (CNV) is the quantitative real time PCR, which evaluates the progression of a PCR reaction in real time and simultaneously quantifies the amount of product amplified. This method is based on the detection of the fluorescence produced by a reporter molecule, which increases as the reaction proceeds, and is characterised by a quencher of fluorescence at the opposite end. The proximity of the reporter to the quencher prevents the detection of its fluorescence. During a real-time reaction, in each cycle the probe hybridises and elongates and the reporter that produces fluorescence that is captured is then released which is subsequently measured for each cycle. The increment of fluorescence is proportional to the increase of product, which is quantified to evaluate gene copy number variations through the co-amplification of a control gene [38].

5. CAH genotype: Phenotype correlation

Several studies have reported high levels of concordance between genotype and phenotype in patients with CAH, however genotype–phenotype correlation is weaker in less severe forms of the disease [42]. As described above, these pathogenic variants are almost entirely correlated with the clinical severity and are well characterised and are associated with distinct clinical forms of the disease. Accordingly, both the classic and non-classical forms of the disease are associated with different genotypes [21]. *In vitro* studies of the expression of the CYP21A2 protein enable the determination of the rate of enzymatic activity that is associated with each pathogenic variant. The majority of CAH patients due to 21-OH deficiency are characterised by compound heterozygotes and there are severe phenotypes of classic forms, which must present two severe pathogenic variants and have no mild pathogenic variants [10, 16, 21]. Alongside there is a genotype of a NC form which has either moderate pathogenic variants in both alleles or one severe mutation and one moderate mutation [38]. The mild pathogenic variant allows for the synthesis of 21-hydroxylase enzyme up to 50% of normal activity, although the severe pathogenic variant does not contribute to any synthesis (**Table 3**).

Variant		% enzyme active	Phenotype
Severe	Large gene deletions and conversions	0%	Classic SW-CAH
	8 bp del		
	E6 cluster		
	p.Gln319Ter (Q318X)		
	p.Arg357Trp (R356W)		
Intermediate	p.Ile173Asn (I172N)	<1–2%	Classic SV-CAH
Mild	p.Pro31Leu (P30L)	20–60%	Non-Classic CAH
	p.Val282Leu (V281L)		
	p.Pro454Ser (P453S)		

SW: Salt-wasting; SV: Simple virilizing.

Table 3.
Genotype–phenotype correlation for the most common pathogenic variants, according to the percentage of enzyme activity.

Patients with the classic form of CAH usually present severe pathogenic variants in both alleles, presenting nil or less than 5% of 21-OH enzymatic activity [23]. The well-known intronic splice site pathogenic variant in intron 2, which consists of the substitution of an A/C nucleotides by a guanine, constitutes a serious alteration, since it causes the occurrence of alternative splicing and an abnormal protein [21]. Many patients present this pathogenic variant in homozygosity with low levels, or even a complete absence of aldosterone, which is typical of the SV form. In turn, patients with the SV form often present only 1–2% of enzyme normal activity, which, despite being low, is sufficient for the synthesis of aldosterone (**Table 3**) [38].

The clinical spectrum of CAH varies widely between the different forms of the disease, however clinical presentation can be particularly diverse in less severe forms. The phenotype is usually predicted by the less severely-affected allele, although the existence of a more severe pathogenic variant in a second allele, rather an intermediate pathogenic variant, can develop into a more severe phenotype [25]. Compound heterozygous for a mild and a severe pathogenic variant has been reported in NC-CAH patients, showing higher basal and stimulated levels of 17-OHP and hyperandrogenic signs when compared with both mild pathogenic variants [6, 62]. Furthermore, CAH carriers are also characterised by higher than normal 17-OHP levels after ACTH stimulation, albeit not as high as the levels registered in CAH patients.

Although there is a relatively high concordance between genotype and phenotype, there are several examples of variability, particularly for moderately affected patients [63]. Both the pathogenic variants designated as c.293-13A/C > G (IVS2–13) and p.Ile173Asn (I172N) result in variable degrees of 21-hydroxylase activity. Those patients who would generally be expected to be SV cases can sometimes be SW, while others can have a NC-CAH-like phenotype [52, 58]. Another example is the p.Pro31Leu (P30L) in exon 1 of the *CYP21A2* gene, which is usually associated with the NC-CAH form, but is also often present in the SV-CAH phenotypes [63]. The lack of correlation between genotype and phenotype is probably the result of an incomplete gene sequencing, particularly in cases where the whole gene sequencing was not performed. The impairment of 21-OH deficiency is responsible for three major types of the disease, representing a continuum spectrum of clinical severity [22].

Familial segregation studies are recommended for a correct analysis of the parental segregation of the pathogenic variants in order to obtain a better understanding of the disease. Pathogenic variants may be placed in opposite alleles (*trans* configuration) or in the same allele (*cis* configuration). In the case of the latter, the individual is not clinically affected. A possible pitfall of PCR-based strategies is that the interpretation of the diagnosis can be complicated, due to the failure to amplify one haplotype, which results in misdiagnosis. The evaluation of flanking microsatellite markers in all family members can minimise this issue and the establishment of a familial segregation pattern is recommended for individuals with homozygous or hemizygous genotypes (i.e., those who have a pathogenic variant in one chromosome and a deletion in the other one).

6. Prenatal diagnosis and treatment

The objective of prenatal diagnosis and treatment of CAH is to avoid genital ambiguity in females and prevent precocious puberty in males, as well as to minimise the psychological and physical aspects related with manifestations of an excess of androgen [39]. Prenatal diagnosis is also of major importance for families at risk of having children with the classic form of CAH, due to the determination of previous carrier status, or due to previous CAH-affected children [39]. Different methods of prenatal detection have been used for several years, such as measurements of 17-OHP in amniotic fluid, or chorionic villus sampling and the molecular genetic analysis of pathogenic variants through DNA that is extracted from chorionic villus cells or amniocytes [27]. These procedures can be informative for fetal gender and carrier/affected status and they can be carried out late on during the first trimester through to the second trimester by the 10th week of gestation for chorionic villus sampling, or around the 16th–17th week in the cases of amniocentesis [39]. The prenatal treatment of this disease involves the administration of dexamethasone to the pregnant woman, starting from 6th to the 7th week of gestation, in order to minimise the effects of genital virilization in affected female foetuses [64]. Dexamethasone is a very powerful glucocorticoid with weak mineralocorticoid activity and is still considered to be a controversial therapy in the prenatal context, as the effectiveness of this treatment is approximately 75%, and the adverse effects for both pregnant woman and the fetus in the long term are not yet fully known [21, 64]. Postnatal treatment can be administered chronically or acutely during a salt wasting crisis and in both cases high amounts of sodium chloride (NaCl) need to be infused, as well as hydrocortisone in an acute case [15]. A careful assessment of the efficiency and suitability of glucocorticoid therapy is carried out by the monitorisation of the urinary excretion of 17-ketosteroids, pregnanetriol, and also plasma levels of 17-OHP [15].

7. New clues at genotyping

A promising aspect that can result from genotyping is prevention of CAH. *CYP21A2* genotyping is strongly recommended in couples with a personal or familial history of CAH who are trying to conceive, in order to obtain a genetic diagnosis of clinically-confirmed cases and prescribe suitable genetic counselling. Although there is a strong correlation between genotype and phenotype, occasionally the genotype interpretation is rather difficult to make due to genetic complexity. In the case of a couple where one of the partners has CAH, the risk of giving birth to an offspring who is affected is dependent on the partner's genotype. If a CAH-homozygous patient with p.Val282Leu has a partner who is a carrier of a CAH pathogenic variant, then the risk of having a child with NC-CAH is 50%. The probability of an individual from the general population being a carrier of a severe pathogenic variant is 1:60 (approximately 1.7%) [22, 24] and the probability of a NC-CAH patient being a carrier of a mild pathogenic variant is approximately 60%, which occurs in about two thirds of cases. In such a case, the risk of having a child with a classical form of CAH is expected to be just 1:600 [62]. Nevertheless, it is understood that the real frequency would be higher, due to the higher carrier frequency in particular ethnic groups.

Therefore, the genotyping of both parents should be a mandatory procedure as part of a prenatal study protocol for couples in which one has CAH [65]. Prenatal diagnosis using nucleic acids circulating in maternal blood (cff-DNA: cell free-fetal DNA) enables gender determination during early pregnancy. By being able to identify the *SRY* gene sequences in maternal circulation, male foetuses do not need to continue to be exposed to prenatal treatment with glucocorticoids, contrary to female foetuses, in which the prevention of genital ambiguity is a concern. Besides determining gender, an analysis of the *CYP21A2* gene by using the most recent massive sequencing technologies for fetal fraction present in maternal blood should be used, however this procedure is very complex and it is subject to a relatively large rate of false positive and negative results.

Traditional invasive methods still provide more confident results, albeit these are usually only performed rather late during pregnancy, which thus compromises decision making regarding the administration of dexamethasone-suppressive treatment during pregnancy when genetic severe forms are identified [66]. Furthermore, Preimplantation Genetic Testing (PGT) in conjunction with *in vitro* fertilisation (IVF) techniques is already a reality, which is designed to avoid the transmission of various diseases. Embryos are genetically analysed by using molecular genotyping and haplotyping techniques and only genetically transferable embryos (i.e., without the disease) are transferred to the woman's uterus, which accordingly stops the transmission of a disease within a family [67].

8. Conclusions

As congenital adrenal hyperplasia is a common autosomal recessive disorder, its incidence in a carrier is higher, particularly in specific populations. The typical symptoms are manifested during the neonatal period, childhood, adolescence, and adulthood, and may lead to an ascertainment bias in favour of the identification of affected females. This is particularly the cases in NC-CAH patients, where the use of 17-OHP measurements tests are not so precise and it is essential to carry out molecular diagnostic studies at *CYP21A2* locus in addition. Genotype–phenotype correlations are of major importance for contributing to an integrated analysis, where specific treatment and genetic counselling also needs to be personalised.

Nomenclature

Nomenclature of *CYP21A2* variants is in accordance with the CYP21A2–002 ensembl transcript, namelly ENST00000418967.6 [NM_000500 from National Center for Biotechnology Information].

Author details

Berta Carvalho[1*], Filipa Carvalho[1,2] and Davide Carvalho[2,3,4]

1 Faculty of Medicine of the University of Porto, Genetics Unit, Department of Pathology, Porto, Portugal

2 Instituto de Investigação e Inovação em Saúde (i3S), University of Porto, Porto, Portugal

3 Department of Endocrinology, Diabetes and Metabolism, Universitary Hospital Center of S. João, Portugal

4 Faculty of Medicine of the University of Porto, Department of Medicine, Porto, Portugal

*Address all correspondence to: bertalc@med.up.pt

References

[1] Campbell I. Adrenocortical hormones. Anaesthesia and Intensive Care Medicine. Elsevier Ltd. 2011;**12**(10):461-464

[2] Robins T. Functional and Structural Studies on CYP21 Mutants in Congenital Adrenal Hyperplasia. Sweden: Karolinska Institutet; 2005

[3] Gonçalves J, Friães A, Moura L. Congenital adrenal hyperplasia: Focus on the molecular basis of 21-hydroxylase deficiency. Expert Reviews in Molecular Medicine. 2007;**9**(11):1-23. DOI: 10.1017/S1462399407000300

[4] Speiser PW. Congenital adrenal hyperplasia owing to 21-hydroxylase deficiency. Endocrinology and Metabolism Clinics of North America. 2001;**30**(1):31-59, vi. DOI: 10.1016/s0889-8529(08)70018-5

[5] Miller WL. The Adrenal Cortex and its Disorders. Brook's Clinical Pediatric Endocrinology. New Jersey: WileyBlackwell; 2009. pp. 283-326

[6] Krone N, Braun A, Roscher A. Predicting phenotype in steroid 21-hydroxylase deficiency? Comprehensive genotyping in 155 unrelated, well defined patients from southern Germany. The Journal of Clinical Endocrinology and Metabolism. 2000;**85**(3):1059-1065. DOI: 10.1210/jcem.85.3.6441

[7] Riepe F, Sippell W. Recent advances in diagnosis, treatment, and outcome of congenital adrenal hyperplasia due to 21-hydroxylase deficiency. Reviews in Endocrine and Metabolic Disorders. Springer US. 2007;**8**(4):349-363

[8] Speiser PW, White PC. Congenital adrenal hyperplasia. New England Journal of Medicine. Massachusetts Medical Society. 2003;**349**(8):776-788. DOI: 10.1056/NEJMra021561

[9] New MI. Extensive clinical experience: nonclassical 21-hydroxylase deficiency. The Journal of Clinical Endocrinology and Metabolism. 2006;**91**(11):4205-4214. DOI: 10.1210/jc.2006-1645

[10] Merke DP, Bornstein SR. Congenital adrenal hyperplasia. Lancet. 2005;**365**(9477):2125-2136. DOI: 10.1016/S0140-6736(05)66736-0

[11] Deneux C, Tardy V, Dib A, Mornet E, Billaud L, Charron D, et al. Phenotype-genotype correlation in 56 women with nonclassical congenital adrenal hyperplasia due to 21-hydroxylase deficiency. The Journal of Clinical Endocrinology and Metabolism. 2001;**86**(1):207-213. DOI: 10.1210/jcem.86.1.7131

[12] Concolino P, Mello E, Zuppi C, Capoluongo E. Molecular diagnosis of congenital adrenal hyperplasia due to 21-hydroxylase deficiency: An update of new CYP21A2 mutations. Clinical Chemistry and Laboratory Medicine. 2010;**48**(8):1057-1062. DOI: 10.1515/CCLM.2010.239

[13] Krone N, Dhir V, Ivison HE, Arlt W. Congenital adrenal hyperplasia and P450 oxidoreductase deficiency. Clinical Endocrinology. 2007;**66**(2):162-172. DOI: 10.1111/j.1365-2265.2006.02740

[14] Green-Golan L, Yates C, Drinkard B, VanRyzin C, Eisenhofer G, Weise M, et al. Patients with classic congenital adrenal hyperplasia have decreased epinephrine reserve and defective glycemic control during prolonged moderate-intensity exercise. The Journal of Clinical Endocrinology and

Metabolism. 2007;**92**(8):3019-3024. DOI: 10.1210/jc.2007-0493

[15] Auchus RJ. Management of the adult with congenital adrenal hyperplasia. International Journal of Pediatric Endocrinology. 2010;**2010**:614107. DOI: 10.1155/2010/614107

[16] Marumudi E, Khadgawat R, Surana V, Shabir I, Joseph A, Ammini AC. Diagnosis and management of classical congenital adrenal hyperplasia. Steroids. Elsevier Inc. 2013;**78**(8):741-746. DOI: 10.1016/j.steroids.2013.04.007

[17] Forest MG. Recent advances in the diagnosis and management of congenital adrenal hyperplasia due to 21-hydroxylase deficiency. Human Reproduction Update. 2004;**10**(6):469-485. DOI: 10.1093/humupd/dmh047

[18] Khan AH, Aban M, Rameez-ul-Hassan N-u-H, Raza J, Jabbar A, Moatter T. Classic virilizing congenital adrenal hyperplasia presenting late: Case series from Pakistan. The Journal of the Pakistan Medical Association. 2009;**59**(9):643-646. PMID: 19750867

[19] Duarsa G. Simple virilizing congenital adrenal hyperplasia: Presentation in a female child with genital ambiguity undergoing Genitoplasty (a case report). Bali Medical Journal. 2012;**1**(3):93-97

[20] Witchel SF, Azziz R. Nonclassic congenital adrenal hyperplasia. International Journal of Pediatric Endocrinology. 2010;**2010**:625105. DOI: 10.1155/2010/625105

[21] Krone N, Arlt W. Genetics of congenital adrenal hyperplasia. Best Practice & Research. Clinical Endocrinology & Metabolism. 2009;**23**(2):181-192. DOI: 10.1016/j.beem.2008.10.014

[22] Trakakis E, Rizos D, Loghis C, Chryssikopoulos A, Spyropoulou M, Salamalekis E, et al. The prevalence of non-classical congenital adrenal hyperplasia due to 21-hydroxylase deficiency in Greek women with hirsutism and polycystic ovary syndrome. Endocrine Journal. 2008;**55**(1):33-39. DOI: 10.1507/endocrj.k07-053

[23] Carmina E, Dewailly D, Escobar-Morreale HF, Kelestimur F, Moran C, Oberfield S, et al. Non-classic congenital adrenal hyperplasia due to 21-hydroxylase deficiency revisited: An update with a special focus on adolescent and adult women. Human Reproduction Update. 2017;**23**:580-599. DOI: 10.1093/humupd/dmx014

[24] Speiser PW, Dupont B, Rubinstein P, Piazza A, Kastelan A, New MI. High frequency of nonclassical steroid 21-hydroxylase deficiency. American Journal of Human Genetics. 1985;**37**(4):650-667. PMID: 9556656

[25] Wilson RC, Nimkarn S, Dumic M, Obeid J, Azar MR, Najmabadi H, et al. Ethnic-specific distribution of mutations in 716 patients with congenital adrenal hyperplasia owing to 21-hydroxylase deficiency. Molecular Genetics and Metabolism. 2007;**90**:414-421. DOI: 10.1016/j.ymgme.2006.12.005

[26] Tardy V, Menassa R, Sulmont V, Lienhardt-Roussie A, Lecointre C, Brauner R, et al. Phenotype-genotype correlations of 13 rare CYP21A2 mutations detected in 46 patients affected with 21-hydroxylase deficiency and in one carrier. The Journal of Clinical Endocrinology and Metabolism. 2010;**95**:1288-1300. DOI: 10.1210/jc.2009-1202

[27] Billerbeck AE, Bachega TA, Frazatto ET, Nishi MY, Goldberg AC,

Marin ML, et al. A novel missense mutation, GLY424SER, in Brazilian patients with 21-hydroxylase deficiency. The Journal of Clinical Endocrinology and Metabolism. 1999;**84**:2870-2872. DOI: 10.1210/jcem.84.8.5937

[28] Billerbeck AE, Mendonca BB, Pinto EM, Madureira G, Arnhold IJ, Bachega TA. Three novel mutations in CYP21 gene in Brazilian patients with the classical form of 21-hydroxylase deficiency due to a founder effect. The Journal of Clinical Endocrinology and Metabolism. 2002;**87**:4314-4317. DOI: 10.1210/jc.2001-011939

[29] Kharrat M, Tardy V, M'Rad R, Maazoul F, Jemaa LB, Refai M, et al. Molecular genetic analysis of Tunisian patients with a classic form of 21-hydroxylase deficiency: Identification of four novel mutations and high prevalence of Q318X mutation. The Journal of Clinical Endocrinology and Metabolism. 2004;**89**:368-374. DOI: 10.1210/jc.2003-031056

[30] Vakili R, Baradaran-Heravi A, Barid-Fatehi B, Gholamin M, Ghaemi N, Abbaszadegan MR. Molecular analysis of the CYP21 gene and prenatal diagnosis in families with 21-hydroxylase deficiency in northeastern Iran. Hormone Research. 2005;**63**:119-124. DOI: 10.1159/000084570

[31] Delague V, Souraty N, Khallouf E, Tardy V, Chouery E, Halaby G, et al. Mutational analysis in Lebanese patients with congenital adrenal hyperplasia due to a deficit in 21-hydroxylase. Hormone Research. 2000;**53**:77-82. DOI: 10.1159/000023518

[32] White PC, Speiser PW. Congenital adrenal hyperplasia due to 21-hydroxylase deficiency. Endocrine Reviews. 2000;**21**:245-291. DOI: 10.1210/edrv.21.3.0398

[33] Lee HH. The chimeric CYP21P/CYP21 gene and 21-hydroxylase deficiency. Journal of Human Genetics. 2004;**49**:65-72. DOI: 10.1007/s10038-003-0115-2

[34] Concolino P, Mello E, Minucci A, Giardina E, Zuppi C, Toscano V, et al. A new CYP21A1P/CYP21A2 chimeric gene identified in an Italian woman suffering from classical congenital adrenal hyperplasia form. BMC Medical Genetics. 2009;**10**:72. DOI: 10.1186/1471-2350-10-72

[35] Blanchong CA, Zhou B, Rupert KL, Chung EK, Jones KN, Sotos JF, et al. Deficiencies of human complement component C4A and C4B and heterozygosity in length variants of RP-C4-CYP21-TNX (RCCX) modules in caucasians. The load of RCCX genetic diversity on major histocompatibility complex-associated disease. The Journal of Experimental Medicine. 2000;**191**:2183-2196. DOI: 10.1084/jem.191.12.2183

[36] Marques CJ, Pignatelli D, Carvalho B, Barceló J, Almeida AC, Fernandes S, et al. Mutational characterization of steroid 21-hydroxylase gene in portuguese patients with congenital adrenal hyperplasia. Experimental and Clinical Endocrinology and Diabetes. 2010;**118**(8):505-512. DOI: 10.1055/s-0029-1237363

[37] Parajes S, Quinterio C, Dominguez F, Loidi L. A simple and robust quantitative PCR assay to determine CYP21A2 gene dose in the diagnosis of 21-hydroxylase deficiency. Clinical Chemistry. 2007;**53**:1577-1584. DOI: 10.1373/clinchem.2007.087361

[38] Parajes S, Quinteiro C, Dominguez F, Loidi L. High frequency of copy number variations and sequence variants at CYP21A2 locus: Implication for the

genetic diagnosis of 21-hydroxylase deficiency. PLoS One. 2008;**3**:e2138. DOI: 10.1371/journal.pone.0002138

[39] Higashi Y, Yoshioka H, Yamane M, Gotoh O, Fujii-Kuriyama Y. Complete nucleotide sequence of two steroid 21-hydroxylase genes tandemly arranged in human chromosome: A pseudogene and a genuine gene. Proceedings of the National Academy of Sciences of the United States of America. 1986;**83**(9):2841-2845. DOI: 10.1073/pnas.83.9.2841

[40] White PC, New MI, Dupont B. Structure of human steroid 21-hydroxylase genes. PNAS. 1986;**83**(14):5111-5115. DOI: 10.1073/pnas.83.14.5111

[41] Lee H-H. Variants of the CYP21A2 and CYP21A1P genes in congenital adrenal hyperplasia. Clinica chimica acta. International Journal of Clinical Chemistry. Elsevier B.V. 2013;**15**(418):37-44. DOI: 10.1016/j.cca.2012.12.030

[42] Yang Z, Mendoza AR, Welch TR, Zipf WB, Yu CY. Modular variations of the human major histocompatibility complex class III genes for serine/threonine kinase RP, complement component C4, steroid 21-hydroxylase CYP21, and tenascin TNX (the RCCX module). A mechanism for gene deletions and disease associations. The Journal of Biological Chemistry. 1999;**274**:12147-12156

[43] Koppens PF, Hoogenboezem T, Degenhart HJ. Duplication of the CYP21A2 gene complicates mutation analysis of steroid 21-hydroxylase deficiency: Characteristics of three unusual haplotypes. Human Genetics. 2002;**111**:405-410. DOI: 10.1007/s00439-002-0810-7

[44] Parker EA, Hovanes K, Germak J, Porter F, Merke DP. Maternal 21- hydroxylase deficiency and uniparental isodisomy of chromosome 6 and X results in a child with 21-hydroxylase deficiency and Klinefelter syndrome. American Journal of Medical Genetics. Part A. 2006;**140**:2236-2240. DOI: 10.1002/ajmg.a.31408

[45] Simonetti L, Bruque CD, Fernandez CS, Benavides-Mori B, Delea M, Kolomenski JE, et al. CYP21A2 mutation update: Comprehensive analysis of databases and published genetic variants. Human Mutation. 2018;**39**:5-22. DOI: 10.1002/humu.23351

[46] Araujo RS, Mendonca BB, Barbosa AS, Lin CJ, Marcondes JA, Billerbeck AE, et al. Microconversion between CYP21A2 and CYP21A1P promoter regions causes the nonclassical form of 21-hydroxylase deficiency. The Journal of Clinical Endocrinology and Metabolism. 2007;**92**:4028-4034. DOI: 10.1210/jc.2006-2163

[47] Tajima T, Fujieda K, Mikami A, Igarashi Y, Nakae J, Cutler GB Jr. Prenatal diagnosis of steroid 21-hydroxylase deficiency by the modified polymerase chain reaction to detect splice site mutation in the CYP21 gene. Endocrine Journal. 1998;**45**:291-295. DOI: 10.1507/endocrj.45.291

[48] Wedell A, Thilen A, Ritzen EM, Stengler B, Luthman H. Mutational spectrum of the steroid 21-hydroxylase gene in Sweden: Implications for genetic diagnosis and association with disease manifestation. The Journal of Clinical Endocrinology and Metabolism. 1994;**78**:1145-1152. DOI: 10.1210/jcem.78.5.8175971

[49] Higashi Y, Hiromasa T, Tanae A, Miki T, Nakura J, Kondo T, et al. Effects of individual mutations in the P-450(C21) pseudogene on the P-450(C21) activity and their

distribution in the patient genomes of congenital steroid 21-hydroxylase deficiency. Journal of Biochemistry. 1991;**109**:638-644. DOI: 1 0.1093/oxfordjournals.jbchem.a123433

[50] Higashi Y, Tanae A, Inoue H, Fujii-Kuriyama Y. Evidence for frequent gene conversion in the steroid 21-hydroxylase P-450(C21) gene: Implications for steroid 21-hydroxylase deficiency. American Journal of Human Genetics. 1988;**42**(1):17-25. PMID: 2827462

[51] Wilson RC, Mercado AB, Cheng KC, New MI. Steroid 21-hydroxylase deficiency: Genotype may not predict phenotype. The Journal of Clinical Endocrinology and Metabolism. 1995;**80**:2322-2329. DOI: 10.1210/jcem.80.8.7629224

[52] Speiser PW, New MI, White PC. Molecular genetic analysis of nonclassic steroid 21-hydroxylase deficiency associated with HLA-B14, DR1. The New England Journal of Medicine. 1988;**319**:19-23. DOI: 10.1056/NEJM198807073190104

[53] Blanche H, Vexiau P, Clauin S, Le Gall I, Fiet J, Mornet E, et al. Exhaustive screening of the 21-hydroxylase gene in a population of hyperandrogenic women. Human Genetics. 1997;**101**:56-60. DOI: 10.1007/s004390050586

[54] Stikkelbroeck NM, Hoefsloot LH, de Wijs IJ, Otten BJ, Hermus AR, Sistermans EA. CYP21 gene mutation analysis in 198 patients with 21- hydroxylase deficiency in the Netherlands: Six novel mutations and a specific cluster of four mutations. The Journal of Clinical Endocrinology and Metabolism. 2003;**88**:3852-3859. DOI: 10.1210/jc.2002-021681

[55] Lajic S, Levo A, Nikoshkov A, Lundberg Y, Partanen J, Wedell A. A cluster of missense mutations at Arg356 of human steroid 21-hydroxylase may impair redox partner interaction. Human Genetics. 1997;**99**:704-709. DOI: 10.1007/s004390050436

[56] Globerman H, Amor M, Parker KL, New MI, White PC. Nonsense mutation causing steroid 21-hydroxylase deficiency. The Journal of Clinical Investigation. 1988;**82**:139-144. DOI: 10.1172/JCI113562

[57] Helmberg A, Tusie-Luna MT, Tabarelli M, Kofler R, White PC. R339H and P453S: CYP21 mutations associated with nonclassic steroid 21-hydroxylase deficiency that are not apparent gene conversions. Molecular Endocrinology. 1992;**6**:1318-1322. DOI: 10.1210/mend.6.8.1406709

[58] Carvalho B, Pereira M, Marques CJ, Carvalho D, Leao M, Oliveira JP, et al. Comprehensive genetic analysis and structural characterization of CYP21A2 mutations in CAH patients. Experimental and Clinical Endocrinology & Diabetes. 2012;**120**:535-539. DOI: 10.1055/s-0032-1323805

[59] Schouten JP, McElgunn CJ, Waaijer R, Zwijnenburg D, Diepvens F, Pals G. Relative quantification of 40 nucleic acid sequences by multiplex ligation-dependent probe amplification. Nucleic Acids Research. 2002;**30**:e57. DOI: 10.1093/nar/gnf056

[60] Krone N, Riepe FG, Partsch CJ, Vorhoff W, Bramswig J, Sippell WG. Three novel point mutations of the CYP21 gene detected in classical forms of congenital adrenal hyperplasia due to 21-hydroxylase deficiency. Experimental and Clinical Endocrinology & Diabetes. 2006;**114**:111-117. DOI: 10.1055/s2005-872841

[61] Bidet M, Bellanne-Chantelot C, Galand-Portier MB, Tardy V, Billaud L,

Laborde K, et al. Clinical and molecular characterization of a cohort of 161 unrelated women with nonclassical congenital adrenal hyperplasia due to 21- hydroxylase deficiency and 330 family members. The Journal of Clinical Endocrinology and Metabolism. 2009;**94**:1570-1578. DOI: 10.1210/jc.2008-1582

[62] Speiser PW, Knochenhauer ES, Dewailly D, Fruzzetti F, Marcondes JA, Azziz R. A multicenter study of women with nonclassical congenital adrenal hyperplasia: Relationship between genotype and phenotype. Molecular Genetics and Metabolism. 2000;**71**:527-534. DOI: 10.1006/mgme.2000.3036

[63] Barbaro M, Soardi FC, Ostberg LJ, Persson B, de Mello MP, Wedell A, et al. In vitro functional studies of rare CYP21A2 mutations and establishment of an activity gradient for nonclassic mutations improve phenotype predictions in congenital adrenal hyperplasia. Clinical Endocrinology. 2015;**82**:37-44. DOI: 10.1111/cen.12526

[64] Dörr HG, Sippell WG. Prenatal dexamethasone treatment in pregnancies at risk for congenital adrenal hyperplasia due to 21-hydroxylase deficiency: Effect on midgestational amniotic fluid steroid levels. The Journal of Clinical Endocrinology and Metabolism. 1993;**76**(1):117-120. DOI: 10.1210/jcem.76.1.8421074

[65] Moran C, Azziz R, Weintrob N, Witchel SF, Rohmer V, Dewailly D, et al. Reproductive outcome of women with 21-hydroxylase-deficient nonclassic adrenal hyperplasia. The Journal of Clinical Endocrinology and Metabolism. 2006;**91**:3451-3456. DOI: 10.1210/jc.2006-0062

[66] Witchel SF. Congenital adrenal hyperplasia. Journal of Pediatric and Adolescent Gynecology. 2017;**30**:520-534. DOI: 10.1016/j.jpag.2017.04.001

[67] Simpson JL, Rechitsky S. Preimplantation diagnosis and other modern methods for prenatal diagnosis. The Journal of Steroid Biochemistry and Molecular Biology. 2017;**165**(Pt A):124-130

Chapter 7

The Surgical Approach in Adrenal Gland Pathology

Radu Mirica and Sorin Paun

Abstract

The pathology of the adrenal gland and the clinical management of the adrenal clinical entities are particularly complex. The surgical approach to adrenal disorders, both in the classic way and especially in the minimally invasive way, is reserved for highly addressable centers and experienced surgeons. The surgical treatment is dedicated to both functional and nonfunctional adrenal tumors, closely following specific criteria. Regarding adrenal pathology, the surgical treatment is indicated for adrenal tumors that secret mineralocorticoid hormones (Conn syndrome), adrenal tumors secreting glucocorticoids (Cushing syndrome), pheochromocytomas, paragangliomas, neuroblastomas, adrenal carcinomas, and metastases. At the same time, non-secreting tumors should be removed as soon as imaging details are recorded an increasing dimensions of these tumors during a short time interval (up to one year). Although laparoscopic adrenal removal became a gold standard procedure in the late 90s, the classic open surgical adrenalectomy is reserved for bulky adrenal tumors and adrenal cancers, but it is overshadowed by possible multiple complications such as lung damage, wound infections, thrombosis, bleeding, etc. The minimally invasive approach, either laparoscopically or robotically, is dedicated to small tumors, with the advantage of rapid patient recovery, rapid socio-professional reintegration, and reduction of complications. Laparoscopic adrenalectomy is indicated in a wide range of pathologies, ranging from Conn adenoma, Cushing syndrome, and pheochromocytoma, to hormonal inactive tumors or other pathologies. The surgical sparing of the adrenal cortex is advised in cases of hereditary disorders affecting the adrenal gland (such as the MEN2 syndrome) in order to avoid primary adrenal insufficiency after the surgical excision. The postoperative evolution must be closely monitored by the anesthetic-surgical team, and the subsequent follow-up must not be neglected. We will discuss the primary surgical indications and contraindications of adrenal gland pathology in this chapter, as well as the perioperative management of specific tumors, surgical approach types, pluses and minuses of various adrenal surgery procedures, surgical technique and tactics, potential complications, and postoperative management.

Keywords: adrenal gland, adrenalectomy, sparing, minimal invasive surgery, surgical approach

IntechOpen

1. Introduction

The pathology of the adrenal gland and the clinical management of the adrenal clinical entities are particularly complex. Surgery for adrenal diseases should only be performed by skilled surgeons in highly addressable centers. The surgical treatment is dedicated to both functional and nonfunctional adrenal tumors.

Regarding adrenal pathology, the surgical treatment is indicated for adrenal tumors that secret mineralocorticoid hormones (Conn syndrome), adrenal tumors secreting glucocorticoids (Cushing syndrome), pheochromocytomas, adrenal metastases, paragangliomas, neuroblastomas, and adrenal carcinomas [1].

In adrenal gland surgery, a multidisciplinary approach involving surgeons, anesthesiologists, endocrinologists, and oncologists plays a key role in patient management. Adrenalectomy is a very frequent surgical intervention with minimal invasive approach in endocrinology surgery [2, 3].

Dr. Lamar Snow performed the first laparoscopic adrenalectomy in 1991, and Dr. Joseph Petelin presented the first description of the procedure in a video at the international symposium of laparoscopic surgery, Saskatoon, Saskatchewan, Canada in August 1992 [4]. In literature, Go H. performed his first laparoscopic adrenalectomy on January 17, 1992, and published it in 1993, after Gagner published his first laparoscopic adrenalectomy in March 1992. Laparoscopic adrenal surgery advanced significantly when Michel Gagner published the lateral trans peritoneal procedure in 1992 [2, 5]. This procedure went on to become the most popular laparoscopic adrenalectomy procedure. The video-assisted approach recognizes three forms, depending on the patient's location and access: first, anterior (trans-peritoneal), second lateral (transperitoneal or retroperitoneal), and third posterior (transperitoneal or retroperitoneal) (retroperitoneal). Soon after, laparoscopic adrenalectomy (after the cholecystectomy) was recognized as the second-best surgical treatment [1].

Transabdominal, transthoracic, and retroperitoneal surgery are the most common approaches to adrenal pathology. To provide a fair control of vascular pedicles' maneuvers therapy, these comprise huge incisions and thorough plan dissections. Postoperative morbidity may vary depending on the surgical technique used to remove the adrenal gland. The development of minimally invasive surgery (MIS) techniques has resulted in significant changes to the majority of surgical operations. The procedure of adrenalectomy is a good illustration of this. The advantages of laparoscopy are completely utilized in this form of approach [2–4].

1.1 Anatomy landmarks

The kidneys and the adrenal glands are in close proximity. The right adrenal is predominantly suprarenal, while the left adrenal is mostly prerenal and medial to the left upper pole of the kidney. An adrenal gland, which is crescent-shaped on the left and triangular on the right, sits above the superior medial pole of each kidney. While the right adrenal gland is frequently supra-renally positioned, the left adrenal gland is typically pre-renally positioned. On the left, between the 11th and 12th ribs, and on the right, between the 12th rib, the adrenal glands are situated in front of the ribs in both regions [2]. The adrenal glands are encased in a capsule that creates septa that convey capillaries into the gland's core [4]. The renal fascia surrounds the adrenal glands, which are surrounded by a significant amount of renal fat (Gerota fascia). The renal fascia's ventral and dorsal layers stretch upward, covering the adrenal glands and attaching to the diaphragm. The renal fascia, which attaches to the diaphragm, as well as big renal veins and arteries, keep them in place. Despite their mobility, the adrenal glands are anchored to the abdominal wall due to their attachment to the diaphragm. That is why hemostasis is challenging because they move in concert with the diaphragm during breathing [5].

For radiological anatomy and also for adrenalectomy, topographic anatomy is crucial. The adrenal glands have a close architecture with several significant anatomical structures, in addition to their intimate association with the kidney. The anterior, posterior, and medial edges of the adrenals are inspected topographically [5].

The renal fat and renal fascia are in contact with the superior portion of the dorsal abdominal wall, which includes the adrenal glands. The 11th and 12th ribs, subcostals muscles, latissimus dorsi muscles, and sacrospinalis muscles are all located adjacent to each adrenal gland, as well as the diaphragmatic crus and lateral arcuate ligament that divide the adrenal glands from the pleura [6].

The right adrenal gland is located 3 mm behind the inferior vena cava and near the celiac ganglion. The gland is not proximal to the renal arteries because of its suprarenal position. It is separated from the pancreas head and duodenal loop on the inferior side by the vena cava, and by the Winslow foramen on the superior side. In contact with the lateral upper region of the anterior face is the inferior medial bare portion of the liver [6, 7].

The inferolateral portion of the anterior side is covered by the peritoneum, which is situated between the liver, kidney, and hepatic flexure. In either a laparoscopic or open adrenalectomy, the peritoneum is open after the movement of the organs, and the right lobes of the liver and gallbladder are brought up while the colon is taken down [8].

The peritoneum of the omental bursa covers the anterior portion of the left adrenal gland superiorly. The peritoneum does not cover the inferior part of the anterior face, despite being close to the medial border of the spleen, the pancreatic body, and the splenic vein and artery behind it. It is connected to the transverse mesocolon on the pancreatic inferior side. The omental bursa and stomach are separated from the adrenal by the pancreatic body. About 7 mm from the aorta, the medial side of the adrenal gland is situated in front of the celiac truncus. The left adrenal gland is near the left renal vein and renal sinus because of its prerenal location [9].

The retroperitoneal region can be reached by separating the splenic flexure and splenic lateral connections, migrating the left adrenal laterally and separating the splenic lateral connections. During the avascular dissection, the veins in front of the adrenal gland, the pancreatic body, and the spleen are mobilized and dragged to the right side. The pancreatic body can also be shifted by opening the peritoneum at the inferior and superior sides of the organ in the bursa omentalis region, especially when the adrenal glands are small. After releasing the gastrocolic ligament, this step is done [8, 9].

The middle and superior adrenal arteries are derived from the aorta, the renal artery, and the inferior phrenic artery, respectively. The lower adrenal arteries come from the renal artery. In addition to other blood vessels, the intercostal and gonadal vessels may also feed the adrenals. These arteries divide into around 50 arterioles under the glandular capsule, creating a rich plexus that needs to be carefully dissected and managed for homeostasis during the adrenalectomy [7–9].

Each adrenal is normally emptied by a single adrenal vein, as opposed to the arterial supply. Controlling this main vein is crucial for physiopathology, especially in malignancies that release excessive hormones. Normally, the left adrenal vein is longer (30mm) and connects the inferior phrenic vein, highlighting the left renal vein after emptying into it. Small (5mm), the right adrenal vein usually drains into the inferior vena cava. Approximately 5% to 10% of persons have accessory veins. These auxiliary veins could directly drain into the left hepatic vein, the right renal vein, or the left renal vein on the left [10].

One lymphatic plexus is located deep inside the capsule, whereas the other is located in the medulla. The adrenal gland produces a vast number of lymphatic channels that run alongside bigger vessels. These lymphatic channels terminate at the lateral aortic lymph nodes surrounding the places where the renal vein drains into the vena cava, as well as the para-aortic lymph nodes close to the diaphragmatic cruris and the renal artery exit. The fact that some lymphatic veins can cross the diaphragm and leak into the posterior mediastinum or the ductus toracicus helps to explain how adrenocortical cancers can spread both locally and regionally. The sympathetic visceral nervous system gives rise to the nerves. The sympathetic celiac ganglia supply the visceral afferent fibers. Nerves and vessels are ligated concurrently during adrenalectomy [9, 10].

2. Indications and contraindications

The majority of adrenal masses are now identified as incidentalomas as a result of the extensive use of ultrasonography and cross-sectional radiological imaging.

Congruent with ESE/ENSAT guidelines, adrenalectomy indications are as follows: functional adrenal tumors, adrenocortical carcinoma, pheochromocytoma, and metastatic tumors. Similarly, patients with unilateral adrenal masses that seem benign on imaging or with adrenal masses that have radiological characteristics that are suggestive of malignancy and have a diameter of less than 6 cm but no imaging signs of local invasion should consider laparoscopic adrenalectomy. For unilateral adrenal tumors with radiological features indicative of cancer and imaging evidence of local invasion, open adrenalectomy is typically performed. The guidelines also suggest surgical removal if the lesion grows by more than 20% over the course of six to twelve months of monitoring of adrenal incidentalomas, combined with at least a 5-mm rise in maximum diameter. Furthermore, surgical treatment should be taken into consideration in a customized manner for individuals with autonomic cortisol secretion who also have comorbidities that may be connected to cortisol excess [11].

Moreover, several studies have reported the outcome of surgical intervention in the potential reversal of autonomic cortisol secretion. Weight reduction, reduced blood pressure, improved glucose tolerance, decreased cholesterol levels, and favorable effects on bone architecture have all been linked to improved metabolic function following adrenalectomy. Cardiovascular benefits in patients with autonomic cortisol secretion were the subject of a recent systematic analysis with adrenalectomy improving cardiovascular outcome and death [12].

An adrenocortical carcinoma poses the biggest risk to a unilateral adrenal lesion with ambiguous imaging features. Surgery is the most crucial therapeutic intervention for adrenocortical carcinoma without metastases. According to recommendations in the guidelines, only referral institutions and surgeons with experience in open and laparoscopic adrenal surgery and who execute more than 15 benign and malignant adrenalectomies annually should perform surgery on patients with this pathology [13].

Hormone-producing tumors have surgical indications regardless of their size. The following are hormone-secreting adrenal tumors for which adrenalectomy is recommended: Cushing's syndrome is caused by an overproduction of glucocorticoids in the fasciculate adrenal cortex, Conn's syndrome is caused by an overproduction of aldosterone in the glomerulosa adrenal cortex, and Pheochromocytomas are caused by an overproduction of catecholamine in the adrenal medulla [11]. Due to pituitary or ectopic ACTH synthesis, adenomas that originate from the reticularis layer of the adrenal cortex and produce excessive levels of androgens and estrogens may infrequently require a bilateral adrenalectomy in Cushing's disease [7].

Nonfunctioning adrenocortical malignancies account for around a half of adrenocortical cancers. Thus, 50% is composed of tumors that secrete 15% cortisol, 10% androgens, 5% estrogens, and only 1% aldosterone, and the remaining 18% of tumors may secrete other hormonal varieties [7]. Malignant pheochromocytomas account for about 12% to 29% of all pheochromocytomas. Lung and breast malignancies, melanoma, renal cell carcinoma, and lymphoma frequently metastasize to the adrenal gland. Adrenalectomy may be required in these patients. The risk of malignancy associated with the size of a nonfunctional adrenal tumor is an indication for surgery. The risk of cancer is roughly 2% if the lesions are less than 4 cm in diameter. Malignancy is 6% more likely in lesions that are 4–6 cm long, and 25% more likely in lesions that are 6 cm long [11]. At the time of diagnosis, 90 percent of adrenocortical tumors have a diameter of more than 4 cm. Most adrenal masses discovered by chance are less than 4 cm in diameter and nonfunctional. Patients who have benign imaging results are not candidates for surgery, although clinical and radiological follow-up is suggested at 6–12 months. Even if that case where the imaging findings are benign, surgical therapy should be considered for each tumor separately since the risk of malignancy increases with the size of the mass [14, 15]. Some disorders, such as asymptomatic myelolipoma or a simple cyst with a diameter of more than 4 cm, may not require surgery [1, 12, 16].

3. Preoperative preparation

Surgical treatment is an option in the management of adrenal masses, respecting the indications mentioned above. In the case of adrenalectomy, the preoperative preparation is determined by the pathology for which the procedure is conducted. The preoperative preparation for an adrenalectomy for a benign nonsecretory or malignant nonsecretory disease is no different than for any other surgery. The condition in which we are dealing with pheochromocytoma, the patient necessitates specific preparation, as outlined in a previously published chapter.

Patients with pheochromocytoma are treated with alpha-blockers, intravascular volume expansion, and beta-blockers (especially if concerns regarding tachyarrhythmia are present) prior to adrenal surgery. Patients may develop substantial hypotension when the tumor is free of vascularization, particularly after dividing the adrenal vein intraoperatively. This necessitates fluid optimization and inotropic support, which may need to be continued in the immediate postoperative period. In addition, mineralocorticoid receptor antagonists, such as spironolactone or eplerenone, are frequently recommended to patients with adrenal incidentalomas and primary hyperaldosteronism. This specific medication should be stopped after adrenalectomy for primary aldosteronism in order to avoid hyperkalemia. Depending on the patient's postoperative blood pressure, other antihypertensives may be discontinued or lowered. Despite successful surgery, older patients and those with long-standing hypertension are more likely to suffer permanent vascular damage and need antihypertensive medication for a long period of time [14]. Furthermore, current endocrine guidelines support perioperative glucocorticoid medication at major surgical stress dosages for patients with autonomic cortisol secretion as part of preoperative care.

Adrenal surgery can be done either laparoscopically or openly. Transabdominal or retroperitoneal approaches can be used for both techniques. The gland can be reached transabdominal or retroperitoneal in either technique [7]. Laparoscopic surgery can be performed in a traditional or robotic manner. With a single port, both ways can be used [13]. The surgical procedure is influenced by the size and also by the kind of the lesion, the patient's general features, and the surgeon's level of experience. Laparoscopic adrenalectomy is really regarded as the best course of therapy for some people [14]. Laparoscopic transabdominal or retroperitoneoscopic surgery has benefits over open surgery in terms of shorter hospital stays, postoperative discomfort, intraoperative blood loss, total 30-day postoperative sequelae, and mortality. Over the past ten years, mortality following adrenalectomy has decreased, with a fatality rate of < 2% [1].

3.1 Adrenalectomy – surgical technique

Furthermore, the surgical strategy is determined by the surgeon's preference, expertise, and knowledge with the procedures. Aspects to take into account include the patient's unique pathological history of abdominal or retroperitoneal surgical procedures, body mass index, tumor size, and location. However, the surgical approach may be impacted by these factors [14].

Normal anatomy is included in the laparoscopic method, and if open surgery is required for special circumstances, it may be done easily [15]. Although the retroperitoneal method allows for direct access to the adrenal gland and requires less dissection and mobilization of other visceral organs, general surgeons find it difficult to master because of a lack of experience. The retroperitoneal surgical approach is also contraindicated in patients with a high body mass index and excessive retroperitoneal fat, as well as those with tumors larger than seven to eight centimeters in diameter. In addition, a tumor near the inferior vena cava on the right side or the aorta on the left may require a difficult retroperitoneal excision. In terms of operating times, blood loss volumes, intraoperative hemodynamic events, rates of morbidity and death, and rates of switching from a minimally invasive to an open surgery approach, retrospective reviews of the literature have shown that laparoscopic and robotic excision of pheochromocytomas are equivalent [9]. The advantages of robotic adrenalectomy also include three-dimensional access, increased wrist mobility for the surgeon, and a stable camera port. Robotic adrenal surgery has certain drawbacks, including rising costs, a slow learning curve, and a lack of tactile input [3].

Patients should be positioned supine on the operating table for laparoscopic transabdominal lateral adrenalectomy. A nasogastric tube and Foley catheter are normally put in after general anesthesia is administered. The patient is positioned in a lateral decubitus position with the afflicted side facing up. A raised arm board is employed, and an axillary cushion is used to support the elevated arm. The superior iliac spine should be the breakpoint for the operating table, and the bed should be bent to expand the working area. The table is bent by around 100–120 degrees in reference to the ground plane to widen the space between the iliac crest and the costal edge. The surgeon and assistant stand side by side and face the patient's front while the monitor is placed at the patient's head side [15].

CO_2 insufflation is conducted after gaining peritoneal access 2 cm inferior to the right/left costal border in the midclavicular line, using either the blind (Verres Needle) or optical (Hasson) trocar. An open approach to the first trocar site can also cause pneumoperitoneum. CO_2 insufflation is usually done with low/medium flow rate of inflation until a pressure of 12–14 mmHg [15]. Between the midclavicular line medially and the anterior axillary line laterally, four 10-mm trocars are inserted 2 cm below the costal margin. Additional ports may be placed if necessary [7], often one 10-mm trocar in the upper epigastric area (to be utilized for retraction - liver for the right side or spleen for the left side).

The first port is often accessed by the midclavicular line. Adrenalectomy is frequently performed through four ports on the right and three to four ports on the left. The inferior vena cava image will remain straight and parallel throughout the procedure as long as the midclavicular line trocar is employed as a camera port on the right side of the procedure (30-degree laparoscope). The two medial ports, together with the anterior axillary line port, can all be used as functional ports. The instruments and ports, on the other hand, can be replaced as needed to give optimal exposure. A liver retractor is normally inserted through the port below the xiphoid process, parallel to inferior margin of the liver. It is strongly advisable to use only a 10-mm trocar in order to facilitate the use of different laparoscopic devices (including suction devices, seal and cut devices, and special clamps). More than 5 cm between the ports should be left to allow laparoscopic instruments to move freely [17–19].

A fourth port is typically positioned laterally on the middle axillary line or medially on the midclavicular line, although adrenalectomy can be performed with three ports on the left side, spaced 5 centimeters apart from the anterior axillary line. The abdomen is examined once the surgeon has entered the peritoneal area to look for any disease and injuries caused by the installation of the port, but because the patient is positioned on his lateral side, little information can be gathered (consequently, it is mandatory for a surgeon to investigate the patient in order not to have any intraoperative findings that can lead to a conversion to open surgery) [19, 20].

For the right adrenalectomy, two working ports are used to insert an atraumatic grasper and an L-hook cautery. If mobilization of the visceral surface of the liver is not successfully achieved by simple upward retraction of liver segments V and VI, a retractor is inserted under the liver, the liver is retracted and the right triangular ligament of the liver is first detached. Thus, the inferior vena cava is reached medially after opening the posterior peritoneum with the cautery, starting from the right triangular ligament of the liver and removing 1 cm from the edge of the liver, thus exposing and dissecting the fascia of Gerota. While the surgeon applies inferior lateral counter-traction on the superior pole of the kidney, avoiding any pressure over the adrenal tissue, the assistant must provide appropriate retraction of the liver in a superior medial way so as not to drain it and to avoid the release of any hormone product into the systemic blood circulation [9, 21, 22].

Normally, the upper medial part of the adrenal is dissected first by the surgical team, unless the adrenal tumor does not invade the lateral wall of the inferior vena cava or if the adrenal tumor is located posterior to the vein. During this dissection, we may use a Harmonic® scalpel (Ethicon Endo-Surgery INC- Johnson & Johnson Medical SPA, NJ, USA), LigaSureTM (Medtronic, Minneapolis, MN, USA), or any other medical sealing and cutting device, preferably 10 mm in diameter, so that enough connective tissue can be trapped to be sealed along with the dedicated vessels.

Using a little piece of fabric, the surgeon can gently move the adrenal gland laterally without damaging it. The adrenal vein is exposed by continuing the dissection from the medial side of the adrenal to the lateral side of the vena cava and is usually a short vein, no longer than 10–15 mm. As it approaches the liver, the right adrenal vein is often visible laterally and slightly below the inferior vena cava. Two clamps are used to transect the lateral side of the wall of the vena cava after circumferential dissection of the adrenal vein. One clip is used to clip the adrenal side, and endoscopic scissors are used to separate it [7, 9, 21]. Sealing and cutting (without clipping) the adrenal vein is also to be performed, if the diameter of this vein is less than 7 mm, according to the technical recommendations of the dedicated laparoscopic instrument.

An auxiliary adrenal vein can be found 2–3 cm above the primary adrenal vein in around 20% of cases and should be dissected, clipped, and divided if present [6]. Alternatively, vascular staples can be used to divide the adrenal vein. The gland's inferior medial side is then dissected. Right adrenal gland's superior medial pole needs special care since there is an artery that has to be ligated or shut off because it supplies the parenchyma. Between it and the upper pole of the kidney is the periadrenal adipose layer of the adrenal gland. It is vital to locate and protect any renal arteries in the higher pole, just like on the left side [13].

The adrenal gland is then pushed up and the dissection is completed on the posterior and lateral sides of the gland as well as superiorly, and during this period of dissection, a particular concern of the surgeon should be not to accidentally injure the adrenal tissue. Otherwise bleeding will occur and it is very difficult to achieve adequate hemostasis with the electrocautery, so it is advisable to use a gauze pad for gentle compression over the adrenal tissue. The gland is removed from the 12-mm port location and placed always in a retrieval bag. If necessary, trocar incisions can be expanded. Incisional hernias should be avoided by closing the port side with a resorbable suture [6, 13, 15]. Many publications propose ligation of the adrenal vein as the first step in adrenalectomy, especially for pheochromocytoma. However, with big adrenal masses, the suitable dissection area for identifying the adrenal vein at the first stage may not be available. As a result, the adrenal vein should be dissected only when it is safe to do so (clearly visualization, good exposure, and no intense traction from the cava wall).

The mobilization of the spleen, which is performed by dissecting the splenic-parietal ligament, is the first stage in the left adrenalectomy surgery unless the division of the left colonic flexure with its proper mobilization is necessary and the first gesture after intraperitoneal video inspection. In the lateral decubitus posture, the splenic-parietal ligament is plainly visible. In order to successfully retract the spleen and expose its posterior aspect, it is recommended to dissect the splenic-parietal ligament starting at the inferior and posterior edge of the spleen, leaving a margin of roughly 2 cm of peritoneum. When the splenic-parietal ligament is separated until it reaches the diaphragm, the fundus of the stomach and the left crus of the organ are visible. Thus, the splenic-parietal ligament is completely dissected, allowing the spleen to be fully mobilized [7, 10].

The splenorenal ligament is then dissected, starting from the posterior portion of the spleen and going to the tail of the pancreas, taking care not to damage this parenchyma. Between the tail of the pancreas and the fascia Gerota, a groove is delineated and an avascular plane is dissected [6]. With the help of gravity, the splenopancreatic block is moved medially out of the operative field, exposing the upper pole of the kidney and the adrenal area, which is brownish in color, not as yellow as the pancreas in the perirenal adipose tissue. The pancreatic tail and spleen are retracted if necessary, using a retractor inserted through a port positioned medially or laterally [16].

Starting on the lateral part of the gland, dissect from the upper to lower adrenal poles, remaining close to the posterior muscle plane. Energy devices are used to separate small arteries encountered during this dissection. The left renal vein is present on the inferior border of the operational field, thus care must be taken to avoid damaging it while the dissection is carried out along the inferior border of the adrenal gland at the same time as the posterior plane, up to the level of the quadratus lumbaris muscle. The left adrenal vein is uncovered by continuing the dissection on the anteromedial side of the adrenal [9, 22].

On the medial side of the gland during this dissection, the left inferior diaphragmatic vein is frequently seen. The left adrenal vein should be exposed by following the left inferior diaphragmatic vein until it reaches it. The medial side of the gland is where it descends. Recognized and isolated is the left adrenal vein. It is longer than the right adrenal vein and empties into the left renal vein (at least 20–30 mm). Contrary to the side of the adrenal gland, which can either be snipped and divided with one clip or divided with an energy device, the side of the renal vein can be cut and split with two clips. Another vein that could need to be cut is the left inferior phrenic vein. If this vein's diameter is less than 7 mm, it can be sealed and severed using a sealing-cutting device, much like on the right side [6, 15].

It is typical to have a tissue tail that extends from the left adrenal gland to the hilum of the kidney. Dissecting the gland from the superior pole of the kidney, right adjacent to the kidney capsule, and all peri-adrenal fat in the specimen are required for an oncologically sound resection. At this point, attention should be paid to locating and safeguarding any superior renal arteries. The last adrenal dissection allows for the "hanging procedure." Pancreas injury should always be considered during dissection using a hook, coagulating scissors, or energy devices in order to avoid a postoperative pancreatic fistula. The adrenal is removed from the retrieval bag using a 10–12 mm trocar [13]. Installing a drain in the adrenal lodge is a solution; however, it is not frequently required. Some authors advise installing a drain there [1, 6, 7, 23, 24].

3.2 Laparoscopic transabdominal anterior adrenalectomy

For adrenalectomy, the anterior laparoscopic route is the least preferable method. The patient is positioned supine, the first trocar is implanted in the umbilicus, and three other trocars are placed in different configurations in the abdominal cavity. However, although it allows different abdominal conditions to be treated at the same time and can be performed bilaterally without changing the patient's posture, the submesocolic technique requires a longer surgical time and more port placements and therefore should be thought about beforehand. It seems to be easier to change the lateral side position of the patient for a bilateral adrenalectomy in the same surgical time [11, 24, 25].

3.3 Posterior retroperitoneal laparoscopic adrenalectomy

Supine positioning of the patient is used to provide vascular access and, if required, place a Foley catheter. The patient is placed in the jackknife position with the table bent to increase the space between the posterior rib edge and the pelvis. The surgeon is on one side of the adrenal gland, while the assistant is on the side that will not be removed. By creating a 1.5-cm incision, 2 cm inferior and parallel to the twelfth rib, cutting through the subcutaneous and posterior muscle layers, and finally reaching the retroperitoneal area, the surgeon can dissect the Gerota fascia posteriorly with his finger [11, 20, 26].

After that, a 12-mm trocar is reinserted into the area, and CO_2 is insufflated at a pressure of 12 to 15 mmHg. A 45 laparoscope is used in place of the 0 laparoscope. On either side of the initial port, two additional 5- or 10-mm trocars are inserted. The adrenal gland and arteries are then located using laparoscopic ultrasonography. The lateral and inferior portions of the adrenal gland are then dissected after the superior pole. The medial dissection is usually done last, after which the veins are identified and separated, as detailed in the previous section on the "lateral transabdominal approach." Feeling the smooth interior surface of the twelfth rib confirms that you are at the right place [7, 13, 15, 26].

Using the Hasson trocar and a direct laparoscopic view, the retroperitoneal region can be reached. Retroperitoneum can be inserted using a finger or a balloon dissector. A 12-mm trocar is then reinserted into this space and the CO_2 is insufflated to 12 to 15 mmHg [7] or 20 to 25 mmHg CO_2 [16]. One 5 or 10 mm working port is inserted medially from the lateral side of the para-spinal muscle to the camera port, and one port is introduced laterally from the middle axillary line to the camera port. A camera with a 30° or 45° angle is utilized [13, 15, 26].

The main markers for this procedure are the para-spinous muscle medially, the peritoneal margin laterally, the peri-renal area, which contains the kidney, adrenal gland, peri-renal fat anteriorly, and the ribs posteriorly. A strong insufflation pressure allows for clear visibility while also compressing any minor bleeding arteries. Hypercarbia and crepitus may occur, necessitating short periods of deflation or reduced insufflation pressures [13, 15, 24, 26].

By pressing down on the kidney and mobilizing the gland inferiorly, the superior attachments of the adrenal might elevate the gland superiorly. Next, the detached, free adrenal vein needs to be located. Utilizing energy-based technology, the remaining adrenal linkages are subsequently removed [15, 26].

3.4 Lateral retroperitoneal laparoscopic adrenalectomy

The patient is positioned the same way as in the lateral transabdominal approach for this type of operation. Similar port placements are used in the posterior retroperitoneal laparoscopic approach as in the posterior retroperitoneal laparoscopic technique. Instead of being on the middle axillary line, the camera port on the anterior side might be placed on the anterior axillary line. The fourth port can potentially be implanted 5–7 cm lower than the anterior port on the anterior axillary line. Important anatomical markers can be used to help with orienting once the pneumo-retroperitoneum has been formed. The fact that the psoas muscle establishes longitudinal alignment and is commonly visible is taken into account by the surgeon. Additionally, the major veins that run parallel to the psoas muscle are visible upon retraction of the kidney anteriorly and upward following medial dissection. Although complete mobilization of the renal hilar arteries is not required following adrenalectomy, the renal artery can be detected by pulse identification. The left adrenal vein needs to be dissected and located via a posterior approach, as opposed to transperitoneal laparoscopy [26, 27].

3.5 Single-incision or single-port laparoscopic adrenalectomy

The single-port approach of laparoscopic adrenalectomy can be done transabdominally or retroperitoneally. Some investigations compared the traditional laparoscopic method to single-port adrenalectomy, finding no significant changes in patient length of stay or morbidity, as well as a minor benefit in cosmetic and postoperative discomfort. There is a lack of data on this strategy, and more research is needed [11, 17, 18, 22, 23].

3.6 Robot-assisted adrenalectomy

Although laparoscopic adrenalectomy has fewer drawbacks than open adrenalectomy in terms of blood loss, pain, hospital stay, and cosmesis, it does have certain drawbacks, such as the need for dexterity, two-dimensional vision, and reliance on a camera assistant. By giving surgeons a three-dimensional magnified view, superior ergonomics, camera control, and multi-articulated instruments, robotic adrenalectomy overcomes the constraints of laparoscopic surgery. Robotic adrenalectomy has yet to achieve general acceptance because of its higher cost and lengthier operating periods. Robotic adrenalectomy can be performed successfully using either the transperitoneal or retroperitoneal technique, depending on the patient's body habitus and the surgeon's skill. It has also been reported to be a viable approach for partial adrenalectomy [19, 24].

3.7 Partial adrenalectomy

In 1983, Irvin et al. [20] suggested cortex-preserving adrenalectomy or partial (or sub-total) adrenalectomy for the treatment of hereditary, bilateral pheochromocytoma in order to retain adrenocortical function and prevent lifetime steroid replacement therapy. The results of partial adrenalectomy utilizing the retroperitoneoscopic laparoscopic approach were published in 1996 [21, 27].

In order to treat minor adrenal masses, partial adrenalectomy is increasingly being used. Therefore, the suggested standard therapy for small benign and hormonally active adrenal tumors may change to minimally invasive partial adrenalectomy [27, 28].

In addition to genetic diseases with a risk of developing numerous adrenal tumors, solitary adrenal masses are now one of the criteria for partial adrenalectomy in bilateral adrenal masses. Particularly in patients with small hormone-active tumors, partial adrenalectomy should be carried out to lower the risk of malignancy. Partial adrenalectomy should not be performed when there are nonfunctional cortical tumors. The surgical reasoning in these cases is determined by the tumor's size and rate of growth at the time of diagnosis, as well as any indication of malignancy. In these patients, a complete adrenalectomy should be necessary [27, 28].

An important consideration in adrenal-sparing surgery is the preservation of the circulatory supply to the adrenal stump. Partial adrenalectomy necessitates the least amount of tissue manipulation and dissection. Studies have shown that patients treated for adrenocortical carcinomas with minimally invasive procedures experience disease recurrence earlier and more frequently due to a greater risk of intraoperative tumor leaking and positive margins. Patients who received laparoscopic resection in Stage 1 and Stage 2 were likewise shown to have worse overall survival rates [24]. In individuals who require lymphatic dissection and adrenalectomy, open surgery should be chosen. For locally advanced malignancies that have invaded surrounding organs or major arteries, the open approach is the best option [9, 13, 24, 26, 27].

Open adrenalectomy is still an option if there are any general or specific contraindications to laparoscopy (a patient cannot undergo laparoscopy if they are unable to undergo pneumoperitoneum, for example), or if there are any specific features of the adrenal tumor that call for a safer procedure, such as the presence of large lesions (12–16 cm in diameter) or the presence of malignant tumor with invasion of nearby structures [27, 28].

The approach used will be determined by the patient's size, location, the likelihood of malignancy, and the surgeon's skill with the various approaches. In addition, the results and morbidity of open adrenalectomy differ depending on the pathophysiology of the disease and the technique used. All peritoneal techniques reduce the risk of postoperative ileus; however, extraperitoneal approaches are associated with significant rates of neuromuscular morbidities, such as persistent discomfort (14%), laxity in the flank muscles (30%), and flank numbness (30%) [2, 29, 30].

4. Postoperative complications

4.1 Postoperative outcomes

Untreated pheochromocytoma has a high rate of morbidity, which is difficult to determine. Cardiovascular reasons can be the cause of death for 71 % of patients, including myocardial infarction, hypertensive heart failure, or hemodynamic instability [18].

The goal of favorable postoperative results with cortical-sparing adrenalectomy is to avoid steroid reliance. The benefit of not using steroids must be weighed against the possibility of recurrence over time. The need for a complete adrenalectomy is determined by a genetic or familial propensity. Cortical sparing adrenalectomies are a suitable option for patients with familial illnesses including MEN 2B, VHL, and/or MEN 2A. Patients with MEN 2A or 2B syndromes who underwent cortical sparing adrenalectomy have a 51.8 percent incidence of recurrence at the age of ten. Moreover, 43 percent of patients who underwent the unilateral or bilateral cortex sparing technique became dependent on steroids. Cortical sparing adrenalectomy is another option for people with VHL syndrome [19].

To prevent recurrence or the development of metastatic illness, which can happen up to 40 years after the tumor was removed, patients with various forms of pheochromocytomas should be monitored for the rest of their lives [17].

There are some relative contraindications to laparoscopic surgery. Many patients can undergo laparoscopic surgery, despite the fact that maybe they had abdominal surgery in the past or they have obesity.

4.2 Contraindication of laparoscopic surgery

In people at high operative risk with cardiopulmonary disease and/or hematological disease, open surgery may be required. Even though previous abdominal surgery and obesity have been cited as relative contraindications for this procedure, many patients in these categories may still benefit from laparoscopic surgery. Therefore, personalized patient management by the surgical team is recommended [24].

4.3 Conversion to open surgery in laparoscopic surgery

There is a small risk when switching to open surgery from laparoscopic surgery, described in some of the studies as about 5 percent [29]. Laparoscopic adrenalectomy should be switched to classic open surgery if there is a macroscopic appearance suggestive of cancer such as invasion into surrounding structures or the presence of suggestive regional lymphadenopathy. Also, intraoperative problems, such as uncontrolled bleeding that cannot be controlled laparoscopically, should be resolved by switching to the classic method if the surgeon fears he cannot control the situation [25].

4.4 Complications of right adrenalectomy

Bowel and vascular injuries, gas embolism, operating difficulties due to adhesions, and obesity are some of the common risks associated with the laparoscopic method. Difficulties may emerge as a result of an incorrect port placement or insufficient mobilization, as well as an incorrect surgical perspective. The right adrenalectomy has a number of particular adverse effects, including damage to the kidneys, liver, duodenum, gallbladder, common bile duct, inferior vena cava, portal vein, right adrenal vein, rupture of the adrenal capsule, and diaphragm injury [1, 6, 13].

4.5 Complications of left adrenalectomy

During port replacement, intra-abdominal organ damage is possible. When a port is inserted, there is a risk of intraabdominal organ harm. Inappropriate port placement, insufficient mobilization, and an incorrect surgical perspective can all lead to difficulties. Some possible adverse effects of left adrenalectomy include splenic artery and vein injury, spleen and pancreatic injury, and stomach injury. Bleeding may occur from poor plane dissection. It is possible to sustain injuries to the left adrenal or inferior phrenic veins. The left renal vein may be divided by mistake, assuming it to be a broad adrenal vein, especially in big tumors. There may be an injury to the left kidney's upper lateral artery, kidney parenchymal injury, gland capsular rupture, and diaphragm rupture [1, 6, 13].

5. Conclusions

In the case of adrenal gland surgery, it is critical to remember that a multidisciplinary approach involving surgeons, anesthesiologists, endocrinologists, radiologists, and oncologists plays a key role in patient management and that surgeon experience and hospital experience both have an impact on the procedure's success. Open adrenalectomy, laparoscopic adrenalectomy, robotic-assisted, and single-incision approaches are only a few of the operations on the adrenal glands that have been recorded in the literature. Surgeons should select the technique with which they are most familiar.

When compared to open surgery, several studies have shown that laparoscopic adrenalectomy is safe, effective, reduces hospital stays, operative blood loss, and wound complications, and has equal long-term outcomes; in fact, it is regarded as the gold standard for adrenal disorders that require surgery. Due to the scarcity of these cases in general practice, the learning curve for laparoscopic adrenalectomy may be difficult. For large tumors and morbidly obese patients, robotic adrenalectomy may offer advantages over laparoscopic adrenalectomy.

In the same way, single port adrenalectomy is technically viable and safe in the hands of an experienced surgeon, but it offers little, if any benefit over other typical laparoscopic adrenalectomy techniques.

Author details

Radu Mirica[1,2]* and Sorin Paun[2,3]

1 Emergency Clinical Hospital 'St. John', Bucharest, Romania

2 University of Medicine and Pharmacy "Carol Davila", Bucharest, Romania

3 Bucharest Emergency Clinical Hospital, Romania

*Address all correspondence to: mirica_rm@yahoo.com

References

[1] Uludağ M, Aygün N, İşgör A. Surgical indications and techniques for adrenalectomy. The Medical Bulletin. 2020;**54**(1):8-22

[2] Go H, Takeda M, Takahashi H, Imai T, Tsutsui T, Mizusawa T, et al. Laparoscopic adrenalectomy for primary aldosteronism: A new operative method. Journal of Laparoendoscopic Surgery. 1993;**3**(5):455-459

[3] Alemanno G, Bergamini C, Prosperi P, et al. Adrenalectomy: Indications and options for treatment. Updates in Surgery. 2017;**69**:119-125

[4] Petelin J. Laparoscopic adrenalectomy. In: Video presented at the International Symposium of Laparoscopic Surgery. Seminars in Laparoscopic Surgery. Saskatoon, Saskatchewan. 1992;**3**(2):84-94

[5] Gagner M, Lacroix A, Bolte E. Laparoscopic adrenalectomy in Cushing's syndrome and pheochromocytoma. New England Journal of Medicine. 1992;**327**:1033

[6] Mirica A, Badarau IA, Stefanescu AM, Mirica R, Paun S, Stefan DAC. The role of chromogranin a in adrenal tumors. Revista de Chimie. 2017;**69**:678

[7] Mirica RM, Ginghina O, Zugravu G, et al. Retroperitoneal functioning paraganglioma - A rare case of secondary diabetes. Chirurgia (Bucur). 2016;**111**(2):170-174

[8] Copãescu C. Suprarenalectomia laparoscopicã. Revista chirurgia. 2008;**134**:25

[9] Mirica RM, Paun S. Surgical Approach in Pheochromocytoma. In: Cianci P, Restini E, Agrawal A, editors. Pheochromocytoma, Paraganglioma and Neuroblastoma [Internet]. London: IntechOpen; 2021 [cited 2022 Jul 28]. DOI: 10.5772/intechopen.96066

[10] Gagner M, Pomp A, Heniford BT, Pharand D, Lacroix A. Laparoscopic adrenalectomy: Lessons learned from 100 consecutive procedures. Annals of Surgery. 1997;**226**:238-246

[11] Maccara D, Mihai R. Surgical embriyology and anatomy of the adrenal glands. In: Clark OH, Duh QY, Kebebew E, editors. Textbook of Endocrine Surgery. 3rd ed. New Delhi: Jaypee Brothers Medical Publishers; 2016. pp. 957-972

[12] Raffaelli M, De Crea C, Bellantone R. Laparoscopic adrenalectomy. Gland Surgery. 2019;**8**(Suppl. 1):S41-S52

[13] Fassnacht M, Arlt W, Bancos I, et al. Management of adrenal incidentalomas: European Society of Endocrinology Clinical Practice Guideline in collaboration with the European Network for the Study of Adrenal Tumors. European Journal of Endocrinology. 2016;**175**(2):G1-G34. DOI: 10.1530/EJE-16-0467

[14] Sherlock M, Scarsbrook A, Abbas A, et al. Adrenal Incidentaloma. Endocrine Reviews. 2020;**41**(6):775-820. DOI: 10.1210/endrev/bnaa008

[15] Gaujoux S. Joint working group of ESES and ENSAT. European Society of Endocrine Surgeons (ESES) and European Network for the Study of Adrenal Tumours (ENSAT) recommendations for the surgical management of adrenocortical carcinoma. The British Journal of Surgery. 2017;**104**(4):358-376

[16] Fassnacht M, Arlt W, Bancos I, Dralle H, Newell-Price J, Sahdev A, et al. Management of adrenal incidentalomas: European Society of Endocrinology Clinical Practice Guideline in collaboration with the European Network for the Study of Adrenal Tumors. European Journal of Endocrinology. 2016;**175**:G1-G34

[17] Gimm O, Duh QY. Challenges of training in adrenal surgery. Gland Surgery. 2019;**8**:S3-S9

[18] Lal G, Clark OH. Thyroid, parathyroid and adrenal. In: Brunucardi FC, Andersen DK, Billiar TR, Dunn DL, Hunter JG, Matthews JB, et al., editors. Schwartz's Principles of Surgery. 11th ed. New York: McGraw Hill; 2019. pp. 1625-1704

[19] Smith CD, Weber CJ, Amerson JR. Laparoscopic adrenalectomy: New gold standard. World Journal of Surgery. 1999;**23**:389-396

[20] Carr AA, Wang TS. Minimally Invasive Adrenalectomy. Surgical Oncology Clinics of North America. 2016;**25**:139-152

[21] Wang DS, Terashi T. Laparoscopic adrenalectomy. The Urologic Clinics of North America. 2008;**35**:351-vii

[22] Tunca F, Senyurek YG, Terzioglu T, Iscan Y, Tezelman S. Single-incision laparoscopic adrenalectomy. Surgical Endoscopy. 2012;**26**:36-40

[23] Machado MT, Nunes-Silva I, da Costa EF, Hidaka AK, Faria EF, Zampolli H, et al. Laparoendoscopic single-site retroperitoneoscopic adrenalectomy: Bilateral step-by-step technique. Surgical Endoscopy. 2017;**31**:3351-3352

[24] Pahwa M. Robot-assisted adrenalectomy: Current perspectives. Robot Surgery. 2017;**4**:1-6

[25] Irvin GL 3rd, Fishman LM, Sher JA. Familial pheochromocytoma. Surgery. 1983;**94**:938-940

[26] Walz MK, Peitgen K, Hoermann R, Giebler RM, Mann K, Eigler FW. Posterior retroperitoneoscopy as a new minimally invasive approach for adrenalectomy: Results of 30 adrenalectomies in 27 patients. World Journal of Surgery. 1996;**20**(7):769-774

[27] Colleselli D, Janetschek G. Current trends in partial adrenalectomy. Current Opinion in Urology. 2015;**25**:89-94

[28] Cavallaro G, Polistena A, D'Ermo G, Letizia C, De Toma G. Partial adrenalectomy: When, where, and how? Considerations on technical aspect and indications to surgery. European Surgery. 2012;**44**:150-154

[29] Long SE, Miller BS. Adrenocortical cancer treatment. The Surgical Clinics of North America. 2019;**99**:759-771

[30] Thompson GB, Grant CS, van Heerden JA, Schlinkert RT, Young WF Jr, Farley DR, et al. Laparoscopic versus open posterior adrenalectomy: A case-control study of 100 patients. Surgery. 1997;**122**(6):1132-1136

Chapter 8

Advances in the Diagnosis and Treatment of Pheochromocytomas and Paragangliomas in the Era of Personalized Genetic Diagnostic

Sofia Maria Lider Burciulescu and Monica Livia Gheorghiu

Abstract

Pheochromocytomas and paragangliomas (PPGLs) are rare neuroendocrine tumors that arise from chromaffin cells. Almost 40% of all PPGLs cases are caused by germline mutations and 30–60% have somatic mutations. The incidence of hereditary syndromes in apparently sporadic cases is as high as 35%. Currently, more than 20 susceptibility genes have been identified, including at least 12 distinct genetic syndromes, with particular clinical features and prognosis. In this chapter, we summarize recent advances in the management of PPGLs from clinical diagnosis to targeted molecular treatment, based on the genetic profile. Classically, patients with PPGLs were diagnosed by sign and symptoms, e.g., hypertension (with or without paroxysms) and headache. Nowadays, about half of PPGLs are diagnosed as incidentalomas or during the surveillance screening in patients with known mutations for PPGL susceptibility genes, familial syndromes, or with a previous PPGL; a high percent of these patients have normal blood pressure. Plasma or urinary fractionated metanephrines remain the major biochemical tests for confirmation. Functional imaging, with a radiopharmaceutical chosen according to the tumor genotype and biology, improves tumor detection (notably for metastases and multifocal tumors) and links to targeted radionuclide therapy. Detecting the germline and somatic mutations associated with PPGLs is a promising approach to understand the clinical behavior and prognosis and to optimize the management of these tumors.

Keywords: pheochromocytoma, paraganglioma, diagnosis, treatment, RET mutation, succinate dehydrogenase mutation, genetic diagnosis, functional imaging

1. Introduction

Pheochromocytomas (PHEOs) and paragangliomas (PGLs) are rare neuroendocrine tumors that arise from chromaffin cells. PHEOs arise from the adrenal medulla, whereas PGLs arise from chromaffin tissues localized outside the adrenal gland, in the paraganglia of sympathetic origin in the thorax, abdomen, and pelvis or of parasympathetic origin in the head and neck region [1].

The incidence of PHEOs and PGLs (PPGLs) is estimated at approximately 2–8 cases/million/year. This percentage may be underestimated based upon the finding that 0.05–0.1% of cases are incidentally detected in autopsy series [2]. Approximately 5–7% of the adrenal incidentalomas are PHEOs [3, 4]. About 80–85% of chromaffin-cell tumors are pheochromocytomas, whereas 15–20% are paragangliomas [4]. PPGLs may occur at any age, and they usually peak between the third and fifth decade of life [4, 5].

PPGLs are usually a benign disease. However, approximately 10–15% of them develop metastases. According to the latest World Health Organization (WHO) classification, all PPGLs are considered to have metastatic potential, changing the previous term "malignant" [6].

PPGLs can appear as sporadic tumors or as part of hereditary syndromes. Almost 40% of all PPGLs cases are caused by germline mutations and 30–60% have somatic mutations [1, 7]. Syndromic presentations, metastatic disease, multiple tumors, bilateral PHEOs, and pediatric PPGLs are clinical features associated with a higher likelihood of a gene mutation [4, 8].

As the incidence of hereditary syndromes in apparently sporadic cases is as high as 35%, in 2017, an International Consensus recommend NGS (Next-Generation Sequencing) to all patients with PPGLs (rather than using one gene at a time) [9]. Nowadays, at least 20 susceptibility genes have been identified, comprising at least 12 distinct genetic syndromes, 15 driver genes, and several new germline and somatic pathogenic variants of genes with disease-modifying potential [1, 7, 10]. These genes are divided into three molecular clusters:

1. Pseudohypoxia cluster 1 (1A and 1B)

2. Kinase-signaling cluster 2

3. Wnt signaling cluster 3.

Between the three clusters, differences in biochemical phenotype, clinical behavior, and long-term prognosis are noted [11, 12].

Cluster 1A-Krebs cycle-related genes (almost 100% are germline mutations, 4–12% of sporadic PPGLs) include succinate dehydrogenase subunits (SDHx [SDHA, SDHB, SDHC, SDHD]) (germline), succinate dehydrogenase complex assembly factor-2 (SDHAF2) (germline), fumarate hydratase (FH) (germline), mitochondrial glutamic-oxaloacetic transaminase (GOT2) (germline), malate dehydrogenase 2 (MDH2) (germline), 2-oxoglutarate-malate carrier (SLC25A11) (germline), dihydrolipoamide S-succinyltransferase (DLST) (germline), and isocitrate dehydrogenase 1 (IDH1) (somatic) [1, 12, 13].

Cluster 1B VHL/EPAS1-related genes (about 25% are germline mutations) comprise von Hippel-Lindau (VHL) tumor suppressor (germline/somatic), Egl-9 prolyl hydroxylase-1 and -2 (EGLN1/2 encoding PHD1/2) (germline), hypoxia-inducible factor 2α (HIF2A/EPAS1) (somatic), and iron regulatory protein 1 (IRP1) (1 case report) [1, 10, 11, 13].

Cluster 2 comprises mutations in genes encoding for a TK receptor (RET) (germline/somatic) genes encoding for the neurofibromin 1 (NF1) tumor suppressor (germline/somatic), Myc-associated factor X (MAX) (germline/somatic), HRAS (somatic), transmembrane protein 127 (TMEM127) (germline), and fibroblast growth factor receptor 1 (FGFR1) (somatic). Also, rare cases with mutations in genes encoding the receptor TKs MET (germline/somatic) and MERTK (germline), encoding B-Raf (somatic) are described [1, 12, 13].

Cluster 3 comprises the transcriptional coactivator 3 (MAML3) fusion gene (gain-of-function event) and somatic driver mutations (0% germline mutations) in the cold shock domain-containing E1 (CSDE1) [1].

Patients belonging to PPGL pseudohypoxia cluster 1 often present at a young age (<20 years of age,) and are predisposed to multiple tumors, recurrence, and metastatic behavior. At least 50–60% of all patients with metastatic PPGL display cluster 1 mutations. Metastatic risk of cluster 2-related PPGLs is low (2–3%), and RET, NF1, TMEM127, and MAX mutations are almost exclusively associated with PHEOs [1, 7, 14]. PPGLs with MAML3 fusion genes were all associated with metastatic disease and showed poor aggressive-disease-free survival [1, 8].

Routine screening in patients with PPGLs is recommended in patients known with mutations in PPGL susceptibility genes, in patients with syndromic features suggesting hereditary PPGLs, and in patients with previous PPGLs, [4].

The treatment options for patients with PPGL are increasingly based on the understanding molecular biology, genetic and epigenetic analyses of the tumors. During the last 20 years, the genetics approach, translational research, metabolomics, peptide receptor-based imaging and treatment, as well as immunotherapy greatly evolved. After the genetic era start, all the clinical, paraclinical features and treatment of PPGLs are reported to their genotype, in an attempt to allow a personalized diagnosis, management, and long-term follow-up of PPGLs.

In this chapter, we summarize recent advances in the management of PPGLs from clinical diagnosis to targeted molecular treatment.

2. Advances in the diagnosis of PPGLs

2.1 Clinical diagnosis

2.1.1 Classical

PPGLs are tumors with a wide spectrum of manifestations, from typically symptomatic disease to asymptomatic disease. Symptoms are present in approximately 50% of patients with PPGLs and are typically paroxysmal. The classic triad of symptoms in patients with PPGLs consists of episodic headache, sweating, and tachycardia [1].

Approximately one-half have paroxysmal hypertension; most of the rest have either essential hypertension or normal blood pressure. Most patients with PHEO do not have the three classic symptoms, and patients with essential hypertension may have hypertension paroxysms. Sustained or paroxysmal hypertension is the most common sign of PPGLs, but approximately 5–15% of patients present with normal blood pressure. Headache is the second most described symptom. Other symptoms include forceful palpitations, tremor, pallor, dyspnea, generalized weakness, weight loss, orthostatic hypotension, polyuria, pallor, cardiomyopathy, panic attack-type symptoms (particularly in PHEOs that produce epinephrine) [1, 3].

PPGLs can produce life-threatening cardiovascular events including acute myocardial infarction, arrhythmias, Takotsubo cardiomyopathy, acute heart failure, or even sudden death [1, 3]. Diabetes or prediabetic states are also a complication of catecholamine-secreting PPGLs. Rarely, patients with a PPGL present with low blood pressure.

Multiple endocrine neoplasia *(RET gene)*—type 2A	Medullary thyroid cancer, primary hyperparathyroidism
—type 2B	Medullary thyroid cancer, mucocutaneous neuromas, marfanoid status, ganglioneuromas of the gut/oral mucosa (Hirschsprung disease)
von Hippel–Lindau syndrome *(VHL gene)*	Hemangioblastoma (cerebellum, spinal cord, or brainstem), retinal angioma, clear cell renal cell carcinoma, pancreatic neuroendocrine tumors or cysts
Neurofibromatosis type 1 *(NF1 gene)*	Neurofibromas, café-au-lait spots, axillary and inguinal freckling, iris hamartomas (Lisch nodules), osseous lesions, optic glioma, carcinomas (breast, lung, colorectal), sarcomas, GIST
SDHx genes	Carney dyad, clear cell renal cell carcinoma, pituitary adenomas (mostly in SDHB, SDHD)

Table 1.
Clinical features of the most frequent hereditary PPGL syndromes.

PPGLs can be sporadic or part of hereditary/familial syndromes, with specific clinical manifestations (**Table 1**).

Head and neck paragangliomas do not produce significant amounts of catecholamines; therefore, they are discovered during imaging studies or by signs of compression or infiltration of cranial or cervical structures, leading to cranial nerve palsies, hearing loss, pulsatile tinnitus, or dysphagia [15].

2.1.2 In the genetic diagnostic era

Due to the increased access to modern imaging techniques and genetic diagnosis, more PPGLs are nowadays diagnosed as incidentalomas or during surveillance screening, either due to genetic risk (germline mutations for one of the known PPGL susceptibility genes) or suspected hereditary syndromes with PPGLs or to a previous PPGL tumor; the clinical picture in these patients may be less suggestive, a higher percent of them having normal blood pressure or being asymptomatic [4, 16]. In a prospective multicentric series of 245 patients with PPGLs, 36% have been incidentally detected, 27% during surveillance, and only 37% due to clinical signs and symptoms [17].

Of note, the likelihood of a PPGL in the first two categories of patients is higher than in those suspected based on the clinical signs [3].

Although most of the symptoms are nonspecific, it has been reported that some signs and symptoms are more evident in screened patients with than without PPGL. Therefore, a score system including specific signs and symptoms has been developed to triage patients according to their likelihood of having PPGLs (−1 to +7 points) (applies to all clusters): [17].

- 1 point for the following specific sign: pallor, hyperhidrosis, tremor (max. 3 points)
- 1 point for the following specific symptom: palpitations, nausea (max. 2 points)
- 1 point for a body mass index (BMI) < 25 kg/m^2 and
- 1 point for a heart rate of ≥85 beats per minute (bpm)
- for obesity (BMI > 30 kg/m2) 1 point is subtracted.

A high clinical feature score (3 points or higher) indicates a 5.8-fold higher likelihood of having a PPGL.

Patients from cluster 2 PPGLs present with higher basic symptom scores and more often suffer from tremor, anxiety/panic, and pallor (related to catecholamine excess) compared with patients from cluster 1 [18].

Some reports suggest that patients with cluster 1-related PPGLs present more often with sustained hypertension caused by the continuous release of norepinephrine into the circulation, while patients with cluster 2-related PPGLs more commonly present with paroxysmal symptoms (so-called "spells") caused by episodic excessive tumoral epinephrine secretion. These spells may be triggered by certain medications, food, beverages (containing tyramine such as red wine and beer), surgery, anesthesia, endoscopy, severe stress, or elevated intra-abdominal pressure (palpation, defecation, pregnancy) [1, 14, 18, 19].

Thus, in cluster 2-related PPGLs, the signs and symptoms are mainly of an episodic nature due to paroxysmal excessive secretory activity. In contrast, cluster 1 tumors, which show low catecholamine contents but higher rates of continuous secretion and less developed secretory control (sustained hypertension) [1, 14, 18].

In RET-related PPGLs, for example, the predominant stimulation of beta-adrenoceptors by epinephrine is presumably responsible for the presentation of episodic tachycardia/palpitations and paroxysmal hypertension rather than sustained hypertension [18].

Interestingly, some patients may be asymptomatic, especially those with small (<2 cm) tumors where there is low catecholamine production or more generally in cases where tumors produce and metabolize but do not secrete appreciable amounts of catecholamines [3].

2.2 Biochemical diagnosis

- Patients with clinical suspicion of PPGLs.

- Patients with incidentally detected adrenal tumors during imaging (incidentalomas, in particular in those with tumor density > 10 Hounsfield units, HU).

- Patients with known germline mutations predisposing for PPGL.

- Patients with syndromic manifestations suggesting hereditary or syndromic PPGL.

- Patients with personal or family history of PPGL should be biochemically tested [1, 3, 4]. There are regional, institutional, and international differences in the approach to the biochemical diagnosis of PPGL.

2.2.1 Classical

The diagnosis of pheochromocytoma is typically made by measurements of urinary and plasma fractionated metanephrines, with negative predictive values >99% at specificities of about 94% [1, 3, 4].

The "gold standard" in diagnosis/screening/follow-up is plasma-free metanephrines (superior to catecholamines, superior to urinary metanephrines), in supine position for at least 20 minutes before taking blood. The most reliable measurements are those made via liquid chromatography/mass spectrometry (LC/MS). A high suspicion for a PPGLs is when we found with more than a twofold increase above reference interval upper cutoffs. Plasma-free metanephrine levels correlate with tumor burden and progression [20, 21].

The adrenergic phenotype is defined by a tumor content of epinephrine that exceeds 5% of the contents of all catecholamines; this can be assessed by measurements of plasma metanephrine relative to normetanephrine, the metabolites of epinephrine and norepinephrine [22].

Adrenergic tumors invariably show additional increases in plasma or urinary normetanephrine; only rarely do these tumors show exclusive increases in metanephrine [18, 22].

Plasma 3-methoxytyramine is useful for detecting the rare dopamine-producing PPGLs [1, 23].

2.2.2 Advances in the genetic diagnostic era

There is a correlation between genotype and the biochemical secretion.

PPGLs of the cluster 1 group are characterized by lower tumoral catecholamine contents, but higher rates of catecholamine secretion per mass of tumor tissue, compared with cluster 2 adrenergic tumors [1, 20, 22, 23].

Increases of plasma-free normetanephrine and/or 3-methoxytyramine with no or minimal increases of metanephrines suggests uniquely and accurately to the diagnosis of a cluster 1 PPGL [1].

Exceptions to this "rule" include the biochemically silent head and neck PGLs and other silent PPGLs with SDHB pathogenic variant, associated with limited amounts of catecholamines in tumor tissue and no minimal increases in plasma normetanephrine or 3-methoxytyramine [24].

The association of cluster 1 mutations with a noradrenergic or dopaminergic phenotype is an excellent example of how catecholamine phenotypes are associated to genetic abnormalities: tumors due to cluster 1 mutations with a noradrenergic phenotype have a higher expression of HIF-2α/EPAS1 than other tumors; they also involve mutations that lead to stabilization of HIF-2α, an important player that blocks glucocorticoid-induced expression of phenyl ethanolamine, N-methyl transferase (PNMT), the enzyme that converts norepinephrine to epinephrine [22, 23, 25, 26].

Cluster 2 is associated with an adrenergic secretion pattern, reflecting a well differentiation of the chromaffin cells in this cluster and, furthermore, a lower tendency to malignant disease in this cluster. The exception to this involves PHEOs due to MAX mutations, in which lack of MAX prevents induction of PNMT by glucocorticoids [1, 23, 26].

Cluster 3-related PPGLs showed the highest chromogranin A overexpression among all clusters [1].

2.2.3 Factors causing misleading plasma MN

Plasma-free MN and NMN levels are frequently elevated in patients with chronic kidney disease, particularly in those on dialysis [27], severe illness narcotic or alcohol withdrawal, anxiety, sleep apnea, essential hypertension, physical exercise. Other substances/aliments that interfere with MN measurements are: nicotine, coffee, sympathomimetics, amphetamine, local anesthetics, lidocaine, cocaine, halothane, MAO inhibitors, bananas, peppers, pineapples, walnuts. There can be seasonal variations in plasma normetanephrine levels with 20% higher levels during winter [20, 28].

2.3 Imaging diagnosis

After the confirmation of the catecholamine hypersecretion, tumor location detection is needed.

2.3.1 Classical

In general, computed tomography (CT) imaging has a high sensitivity (around 100%) but a low specificity (50%) for the screening of PHEOs. It has the highest screening sensitivity if in native phase, the tumor has >10 Hounsfield units (HU) [29].

On the other hand, magnetic resonance imaging (MRI) has a higher sensitivity for head and neck and sympathetic PGLs, compared with CT. MRI is overall preferable for children and long-term follow-up of children and adults [30].

Regarding metastatic PPGLs, CT scan is superior to MRI for lung metastases, whereas MRI is superior to CT for liver metastases [29, 30].

Scintigraphy. 123/131I- meta-iodobenzylguanidine (MIBG) is the most specific radiopharmaceutical for PPGLs (specificity>95%); its sensitivity is decreased in small tumors and/or those associated with SDHx mutations [1, 30, 31].

2.3.2 Advances in the genetic diagnostic era

Functional imaging is recommended for presurgery staging of PHEO ≥5 cm for staging of metastatic/multifocal disease and after surgery of a (sympathetic) PGL or of metastatic/multifocal disease, and it is optional in follow-up in adult SDHx mutation carriers [1, 31].

According to the most recently published guideline for functional imaging of PPGLs, the most sensitive imaging method for cluster 1A SDHx-related disease is functional imaging with somatostatin receptor analogs (SSA) positron emission tomography-computed tomography ([68Ga]-DOTA-SSA PET/CT) with a sensitivity of 94–100% [31–33].

[68Ga]-DOTA-SSA PET/CT is the most sensitive imaging modality in the diagnosis and screening of cluster 1A SDHx-related PPGLs (mostly PGLs), since these tumors strongly express the somatostatin receptor 2 (SSTR2). In contrast, cluster 1B VHL/EPAS1-related PPGLs (specifically PHEOs) show stronger expression of the L-type amino-acid transporter and less SSTR2 expression. Therefore, [18F] FDOPA PET/CT is more sensitive than [68Ga]-DOTA-SSA PET/CT for these patients. Due to cluster 2-related tumors intra-adrenally located (exceptions, HRAS- and FGFR1-related PGLs in the Chinese population), anatomic abdominal imaging with CT or MRI is usually sufficient for tumor localization [1, 31–34].

If there are inconclusive results on anatomic imaging (e.g., very small tumors, multifocality, distorted anatomy), PHEOs ≥5 cm, or for staging of metastatic disease, the most sensitive functional imaging method for all cluster 2-related PHEOs (>1 cm) is [18F] FDOPA PET/CT [35].

For the cluster 3, the most sensitive functional imaging modality is unknown [1].

2.4 Treatment

For locoregional disease, surgery should always be the first-line therapy, whenever possible. Minimally invasive adrenalectomy is the preferred surgical standard [36].

Although cortical-sparing surgery is associated with development of recurrent disease in about 13% of patients with germline mutations in RET or VHL, this is not associated with decreased survival and can be considered for less aggressive PPGLs. Adrenal-sparing surgery should not be favored over total adrenalectomy in most cluster 1 tumors, due to a high risk of recurrence and metastatic spread, particularly SDHB-mutant tumors [4, 36].

Current recommendations from the US Endocrine Society Practice Guideline and the Working Group on Endocrine Hypertension of the European Society of Hypertension agree that alpha-adrenoceptor blockade should be given for 7–14 days before surgery [3, 4]. There is no specific consensus on blood pressure and heart rate targets; however, it is recommended to reach a seated blood pressure target <130/80 mmHg [4, 37, 38].

The most frequently used drugs are the nonselective and noncompetitive alpha-1/2-adrenoceptor blocker phenoxybenzamine [4, 37, 38].

The tyrosine hydroxylase inhibitor metyrosine, which inhibits catecholamine synthesis, can additionally help to prevent pre- and intraoperative hemodynamic instability when given in combination with phenoxybenzamine. The combination treatment reduces blood pressure fluctuations [38, 39].

The mortality rate for PPGL surgical treatment has decreased from about 40% in the past to 0–3% in contemporary series, probably as a result of better preoperative treatment and surgical techniques [1, 40].

3. Special considerations for metastatic disease

PPGL-related malignancy is defined as the presence of distant metastases in non-chromaffin tissues (e.g., bone and lymph nodes) [41]. Approximately 10%–15% of PHEOs and 35–40% of PGLs develop metastases [42].

The metastatic potential of a PPGL is evaluated based on tumor size (≥5 cm), extra-adrenal location, a dopaminergic phenotype (e.g., plasma methoxytyramine more than threeold above the upper reference limit), high Ki-67 index, the presence of a *SDHB* mutation [1, 8]. Histological scores are more reliable in ruling out than in predicting a malignant behavior: *Pheochromocytoma of the Adrenal Gland Score* (PASS) < 4 and *Grading of Adrenal Pheochromocytoma and Paraganglioma* (GAPP) score < 3 [1, 43, 44]. A thorough genetic testing is useful in appreciating the metastatic risk.

At least 50–60% of all patients with metastatic PPGL carry cluster 1 mutations. In a retrospective study investigating 169 patients, 50% of all patients with metastatic disease had cluster 1 tumors (42% SDHB-related tumors), only 4% had cluster 2 tumors, and 46% had apparently sporadic disease [1, 43, 45].

Overall, the highest metastatic risk is reported for SDHB (35–75%), SDHA (30–66%), and HIF2A/EPAS1 mutation carriers (>30%). (1,33,34) Moreover, there also seems to be an increased metastatic risk for patients with FH mutations, while an intermediate risk (15–29%) has been shown for SDHD mutation carriers and an intermediate-to-low risk for SDHC and VHL (5–8%) mutation carriers [1, 42, 45].

Metastatic risk of cluster 2-related PPGLs is low, and RET, NF1, TMEM127, and MAX mutations are almost exclusively associated with PHEOs [43]. MEN2B is associated with a higher metastatic risk compared with MEN2A. The metastatic risk of NF1-related PHEOs is also low (2–12%) [1, 46].

Cluster 3 PPGLs were all associated with metastatic disease and showed poor aggressive-disease-free survival (e.g., a short time until the occurrence of either distant metastases, local recurrence, or positive regional lymph nodes [1].

There are practiced standards of therapy for metastatic PPGLs including chemotherapy (cyclophosphamide, vincristine, and dacarbazine [CVD] scheme, or temozolomide monotherapy), radionuclide therapy ([131I]-MIBG, [177Lu]-DOTATATE), tyrosine kinase inhibitors (TKIs) (sunitinib, cabozantinib), and immunotherapy [47–49].

There are some points to follow about metabolic activity of these tumors before addressing a specific therapy:

- positivity on [123I]-MIBG scan for low or high-specific-activity [131I]-MIBG (expressing the norepinephrine transporter system, less likely positive for SDHx-mutated PPGLs).
- 68Ga-DOTATATE scan for [177Lu] DOTATATE therapy (expressing SSTR2, particularly SDHx-mutated PPGLs),
- PD-L1 status for pembrolizumab, demethylating agents (especially for SDHx-mutated tumors), possibly HIF-2α inhibitors (particularly for cluster 1 PPGLs) poly (ADP-ribose) polymerase (PARP) inhibitors together with temozolomide (specifically for SDHx-mutated tumors) [46–48, 50–52].

Additionally, antiresorptive therapies, such as bisphosphonates and denosumab, are administered in the case of large and numerous bone metastases [38].

For Cluster 2-specific there are some indications for systemic therapy approaches, such as: [131I] MIBG therapy; kinase signaling pathway–related TKIs (sunitinib, cabozantinib, LOXO-292, lenvatinib, axitinib) and other specific targeted signaling pathway inhibitors alone and in combination (PI3K/AKT/mTORC1 inhibitors and RAF/MEK/ERK inhibitors) [50–53].

4. Follow-up in patients with PPGL

In general, every patient with any of the following criteria should undergo lifelong follow-up: [1, 4].

- germline mutation predisposing for PPGL.
- history of paraganglioma.
- age < 20 years at initial diagnosis.
- tumor size ≥5 cm.
- multiple or recurrent PPGLs.
- noradrenergic/dopaminergic phenotype.

Children with an initial diagnosis of SDHx mutation should firstly undergo a clinical examination including blood pressure measurements, plasma-free normetanephrine and 3-methoxytyramine (or urinary normetanephrine), and MRI (base of the skull to pelvis) [54, 55].

After negative initial screening, a clinical evaluation and blood pressure measurement annually, hormonal samples every 2 years, and an MRI (base of the skull to pelvis) every 2–3 years are recommended. Usually, after initial screening, MRI can be performed without gadolinium enhancement, but preferably with diffusion-weighted imaging for maximal sensitivity [1, 4, 55].

For adults, the similar situation is recommended-lifelong follow-up, apart from more frequent biochemistry every year (plasma is preferred, including plasma measurements of 3-methoxytyramine and no consensus for chromogranin A). In adults, initial screening should include functional imaging (PET/CT), but there is no recommendation for alternating MRI and PET/CT during follow-up [4, 55].

For patients with a history of an SDHA/B PPGL (highest metastatic risk), biochemistry every 6 months to 1 year and imaging every 1–2 years are reasonable [4, 41, 55].

For patients with a history of an SDHC/D/AF2- or VHL-related PPGL with a lower metastatic risk, biochemistry every year and imaging intervals of 2–3 years are sufficient [4, 54].

For asymptomatic RET mutation carriers, every year follow-up for PHEOs including clinical investigation and hormonal samples should begin between 11 and 16 years of age—depending on the high or moderate risk for PHEOs specific to the codon involved in RET mutation (always consider the risk of medullary thyroid carcinoma and primary hyperparathyroidism) [1, 4].

Patients with a history of an RET-related PHEO should have a lifelong follow-up with yearly clinical investigation and hormonal sampling; for patients with high and moderate risk for PHEOs (depending on the specific RET mutation), follow-up may include abdominal/pelvic MRI every 5 years [1, 4, 54].

Despite a rather low metastatic risk of NF1-related PHEOs, most recently published guidelines recommend the initiation of a biochemical screening of asymptomatic NF1 mutation carriers every 3 years from the age of 10 to 14 years [1, 4, 22].

For each patient with first diagnosis of a cluster 2-related PPGL $\geq$5 cm, a chest CT is recommended for exclusion of metastatic disease; however, this is unnecessary in the long-life follow-up of these mutation carriers because cluster 2-related diseases are related to a low metastatic risk and almost exclusively adrenal location of the tumor [1, 4, 22].

New discovered genes in the last 5 years: CSDE1(somatic), H3F3A(somatic), UBTFMAML3(somatic), IRP1(somatic), SLC25A11(somatic), DLST (germline), MERTK (somatic), MET (somatic and germline), FGFR1(somatic), SUCLG2(somatic) [7].

5. Final considerations

Cluster-specific management regarding patient education, diagnostics (biochemistry, imaging), and follow-up are already widely acknowledged. Cluster-specific, genetically driven therapy requiring NGS of individual tumors may be an essential part of the management of these tumors in the future.

The ongoing PROSPHEO registry trial (NCT03344016), together with novel artificial intelligence approaches, might be able to answer the question as to the optimal follow-up for PPGL patients and aid in achieving the goal of preventing metastatic spread and death from PPGLs [1].

In conclusion, PPGLs are rare tumors with unique molecular and phenotypic landscapes. Diagnosing the germline and somatic mutations associated with PPGLs is a promising approach to understand the clinical behavior and prognosis and to personalize and thus optimize the management of these tumors.

Conflicts of interest

The authors declare no conflicts of interest relevant to this manuscript.

Author details

Sofia Maria Lider Burciulescu[1,2] and Monica Livia Gheorghiu[1,2*]

1 Carol Davila University of Medicine and Pharmacy, Bucharest, Romania

2 C.I. Parhon National Institute of Endocrinology, Bucharest, Romania

*Address all correspondence to: monicagheorghiu@yahoo.com

References

[1] Nölting S, Bechmann N, Taieb D, Beuschlein F, Fassnacht M, Kroiss M, et al. Personalized management of pheochromocytoma and paraganglioma. Endocrine Reviews. 2022;**43**(2):199-239. DOI: 10.1210/endrev/bnab045

[2] Aygun N, Uludag M. Pheochromocytoma and paraganglioma: From epidemiology to clinical findings. Sisli Etfal Hastan Tip Bulteni. 2020;**54**(2):159-168. DOI: 10.14744/SEMB.2020.18794

[3] Lenders JWM, Kerstens MN, Amar L, et al. Genetics, diagnosis, management and future directions of research of phaeochromocytoma and paraganglioma: A position statement and consensus of the working group on endocrine hypertension of the European Society of Hypertension. Journal of Hypertension. 2020;**38**(8):1443-1456. DOI: 10.1097/HJH.0000000000002438

[4] Lenders JW, Duh QY, Eisenhofer G, et al. Endocrine Society. Pheochromocytoma and paraganglioma: An Endocrine Society clinical practice guideline. The Journal of Clinical Endocrinology and Metabolism. 2014;**99**(6):1915-1942. DOI: 10.1210/jc.2014-1498

[5] Gheorghiu ML, Hortopan D, Dumitrascu A, Caragheorgheopol A, Stefanescu A, Trifanescu R, et al. Age-related endocrine tumors: Non-functioning adrenal tumors as compared to pituitary adenomas. Acta Endo (Buc). 2009;**5**:371-384. DOI: 10.4183/aeb.2009.371

[6] Lam AK. Update on adrenal tumours in 2017 World Health Organization (WHO) of endocrine tumours. Endocrine Pathology. 2017;**28**(3):213-227

[7] Jhawar S, Arakawa Y, Kumar S, Varghese D, Kim YS, Roper N, et al. New insights on the genetics of pheochromocytoma and paraganglioma and its clinical implications. Cancers. 2022;**14**(3):594. DOI: 10.3390/cancers14030594

[8] Fassnacht M, Assie G, Baudin E, et al. Adrenocortical carcinomas and malignant phaeochromocytomas: ESMO-EURACAN clinical practice guidelines for diagnosis, treatment and follow-up. Annals of Oncology. 2020;**31**(11):1476-1490. DOI: 10.1016/j.annonc.2020.08.2099

[9] NGS in PPGL (NGSnPPGL) Study Group, Toledo RA, Burnichon N, Cascon A, Benn DE, Bayley JP, et al. Consensus statement on next-generation-sequencing-based diagnostic testing of hereditary phaeochromocytomas and paragangliomas. Nature Reviews. Endocrinology. 2017;**13**(4):233-247. DOI: 10.1038/nrendo.2016.185

[10] Fishbein L, Leshchiner I, Walter V, et al. Cancer genome atlas research network. Comprehensive molecular characterization of pheochromocytoma and paraganglioma. Cancer Cell. 2017;**31**(2):181-193. DOI: 10.1016/j.ccell.2017.01.001

[11] Jochmanova I, Pacak K. Genomic landscape of pheochromocytoma and paraganglioma. Trends Cancer. 2018;**4**(1):6-9. DOI: 10.1016/j.trecan.2017.11.001

[12] Gieldon L, William D, Hackmann K, et al. Optimizing genetic workup in pheochromocytoma and paraganglioma by integrating diagnostic and research approaches. Cancers (Basel). 2019;**11**(6). DOI: 10.3390/cancers11060809

[13] Luchetti A, Walsh D, Rodger F, et al. Profiling of somatic mutations in phaeochromocytoma and paraganglioma by targeted next generation sequencing analysis. International Journal of Endocrinology. 2015;**2015**:138573. DOI: 10.1155/2015/138573

[14] Timmers HJ, Kozupa A, Eisenhofer G, et al. Clinical presentations, biochemical phenotypes, and genotype-phenotype correlations in patients with succinate dehydrogenase subunit B-associated pheochromocytomas and paragangliomas. The Journal of Clinical Endocrinology and Metabolism. 2007;**92**(3):779-786

[15] Taieb D, Kaliski A, Boedeker CC, Martucci V, Fojo T, Adler JR, et al. Current approaches and recent developments in the management of head and neck paragangliomas. Endocrine Reviews. 2014;**35**:795-819

[16] Plouin PF, Amar L, Dekkers OM, et al. European Society of Endocrinology Clinical Practice Guideline for long-term follow-up of patients operated on for a phaeochromocytoma or a paraganglioma. European Journal of Endocrinology. 2016;**174**(5):G1-G10. DOI: 10.1530/EJE-16-0033

[17] Geroula A, Deutschbein T, Langton K, Masjkur J, Pamporaki C, Peitzsch M, et al. Pheochromocytoma and paraganglioma: Clinical feature-based disease probability in relation to catecholamine biochemistry and reason for disease suspicion. European Journal of Endocrinology. 2019;**181**(4):409-420. DOI: 10.1530/EJE-19-0159

[18] Eisenhofer G, Huynh TT, Elkahloun A, et al. Differential expression of the regulated catecholamine secretory pathway in different hereditary forms of pheochromocytoma. American Journal of Physiology. Endocrinology and Metabolism. 2008;**295**(5):E1223-E1233. DOI: 10.1152/ajpendo.90591.2008

[19] Paul Robertson R. DeGroot's Endocrinology. 8th ed. Philadelphia: Elsevier; 2021

[20] Lenders JW, Pacak K, Walther MM, et al. Biochemical diagnosis of pheochromocytoma: Which test is best? Journal of the American Medical Association. 2002;**287**(11):1427-1434. DOI: 10.1001/jama.287.11.1427

[21] Weismann D, Peitzsch M, Raida A, et al. Measurements of plasma metanephrines by immunoassay vs liquid chromatography with tandem mass spectrometry for diagnosis of pheochromocytoma. European Journal of Endocrinology. 2015;**172**(3):251-260. DOI: 10.1530/EJE-14-0730

[22] Eisenhofer G, Klink B, Richter S, Lenders JW, Robledo M. Metabologenomics of phaeochromocytoma and paraganglioma: An integrated approach for personalised biochemical and genetic testing. Clinical Biochemistry Review. 2017;**38**(2):69-100

[23] Eisenhofer G, Lenders JW, Linehan WM, Walther MM, Goldstein DS, Keiser HR. Plasma normetanephrine and metanephrine for detecting pheochromocytoma in von Hippel-Lindau disease and multiple endocrine neoplasia type 2. The New England Journal of Medicine. 1999;**340**(24):1872-1879. DOI: 10.1056/NEJM199906173402404

[24] Timmers HJ, Pacak K, Huynh TT, et al. Biochemically silent abdominal paragangliomas in patients with mutations in the succinate dehydrogenase subunit B gene. The Journal of Clinical Endocrinology and Metabolism. 2008;**93**(12):4826-4832. DOI: 10.1210/jc.2008-1093

[25] Eisenhofer G, Lenders JW, Goldstein DS, et al. Pheochromocytoma catecholamine phenotypes and prediction of tumor size and location by use of plasma free metanephrines. Clinical Chemistry. 2005;**51**(4):735-744. DOI: 10.1373/clinchem.2004.045484

[26] Eisenhofer G, Deutschbein T, Constantinescu G, et al. Plasma metanephrines and prospective prediction of tumor location, size and mutation type in patients with pheochromocytoma and paraganglioma. Clinical Chemistry and Laboratory Medicine. 2020;**59**(2):353-363. DOI: 10.1515/cclm-2020-0904

[27] Niculescu DA, Ismail G, Poiana C. Plasma free Metanephrine and normetanephrine levels are increased in patients with chronic kidney disease. Endocrine Practice. 2014;**20**(2):139-144. DOI: 10.4158/EP13251.OR

[28] Gardner D. Dolores Shoback Greenspan's Basic and Clinical Endocrinology. Tenth ed. California, San Francisco: Lange; 2018

[29] Buitenwerf E, Berends AMA, van Asselt ADI, et al. Diagnostic accuracy of computed tomography to exclude pheochromocytoma: A systematic review, meta-analysis, and cost analysis. Mayo Clinic Proceedings. 2019;**94**(10):2040-2052. DOI: 10.1016/j.mayocp.2019.03.030

[30] Daniel E, Jones R, Bull M, Newell-Price J. Rapid-sequence MRI for long-term surveillance for paraganglioma and phaeochromocytoma in patients with succinate dehydrogenase mutations. European Journal of Endocrinology. 2016;**175**(6):561-570. DOI: 10.1530/EJE-16-0595

[31] Taïeb D, Jha A, Treglia G, Pacak K. Molecular imaging and radionuclide therapy of pheochromocytoma and paraganglioma in the era of genomic characterization of disease subgroups. Endocrine-Related Cancer. 2019;**26**(11):R627-R652. DOI: 10.1530/ERC-19-0165

[32] Gild ML, Naik N, Hoang J, et al. Role of DOTATATE-PET/CT in preoperative assessment of phaeochromocytoma and paragangliomas. Clinical Endocrinology. 2018;**89**(2):139-147. DOI: 10.1111/cen.13737

[33] Jha A, Ling A, Millo C, et al. Superiority of 68Ga-DOTATATE PET/CT to other functional and anatomic imaging modalities in the detection of SDHD-related pheochromocytoma and paraganglioma–a comparative prospective study. Journal of Nuclear Medicine. 2018;**59**(supplement 1):46. DOI: 10.1158/1078-0432.CCR-14-2751

[34] Janssen I, Blanchet EM, Adams K, et al. Superiority of [68Ga]-DOTATATE PET/CT to other functional imaging modalities in the localization of SDHB-associated metastatic pheochromocytoma and paraganglioma. Clinical Cancer Research. 2015;**21**(17):3888-3895. DOI: 10.1158/1078-0432.CCR-14-2751

[35] Taïeb D, Hicks RJ, Hindié E, et al. European Association of Nuclear Medicine Practice Guideline/Society of Nuclear Medicine and Molecular Imaging procedure standard 2019 for radionuclide imaging of phaeochromocytoma and paraganglioma. European Journal of Nuclear Medicine and Molecular Imaging. 2019;**46**(10):2112-2137

[36] Castinetti F, Qi XP, Walz MK, et al. Outcomes of adrenal-sparing surgery or total adrenalectomy in phaeochromocytoma associated with multiple endocrine neoplasia type 2: An international retrospective

population-based study. The Lancet Oncology. 2014;**15**(6):648-655. DOI: 10.1016/S1470-2045(14)70154-8

[37] Berends AMA, Kerstens MN, Lenders JWM, Timmers H. Approach to the patient: Perioperative management of the patient with pheochromocytoma or sympathetic paraganglioma. The Journal of Clinical Endocrinology and Metabolism. 2020;**105**(9):3088-3103. DOI: 10.1210/clinem/dgaa441

[38] Uslar T, San Francisco IF, Olmos R, Macchiavelo S, Zuñiga A, Rojas P, et al. Clinical presentation and perioperative Management of Pheochromocytomas and Paragangliomas: A 4-decade experience. J Endocr Soc. 2021;**5**(10): bvab073

[39] Steinsapir J, Carr AA, Prisant LM, Bransome ED Jr. Metyrosine and pheochromocytoma. Archives of Internal Medicine. 1997;**157**(8):901-906

[40] Patel D. Surgical approach to patients with pheochromocytoma. Gland Surgery. 2020;**9**(1):32-42

[41] Hescot S, Curras-Freixes M, Deutschbein T, et al. European network for the study of adrenal Tumors (ENS@T). Prognosis of malignant pheochromocytoma and paraganglioma (MAPP-Prono Study): A European network for the study of adrenal Tumors retrospective study. The Journal of Clinical Endocrinology and Metabolism. 2019;**104**(6):2367-2374. DOI: 10.1210/jc.2018-01968

[42] Leijon H, Remes S, Hagström J, Louhimo J, Mäenpää H, Schalin-Jäntti C, et al. Variable somatostatin receptor subtype expression in 151 primary pheochromocytomas and paragangliomas. Human Pathology. 2019;**86**:66-75. DOI: 10.1016/j.humpath.2018.11.020

[43] King KS, Prodanov T, Kantorovich V, Fojo T, Hewitt JK, Zacharin M, et al. Metastatic pheochromocytoma / paraganglioma related to primary tumor development in childhood or adolescence: Significant link to SDHB mutations. Journal of Clinical Oncology. 2011;**29**(31):4137-4142. DOI: 10.1200/JCO.2011.34.6353

[44] Kimura N, Takayanagi R, Takizawa N, et al. Phaeochromocytoma Study Group in Japan. Pathological grading for predicting metastasis in phaeochromocytoma and paraganglioma. Endocrine-Related Cancer. 2014;**21**(3):405-414

[45] Crona J, Lamarca A, Ghosal S, Welin S, Skogseid B, Pacak K. Genotype-phenotype correlations in pheochromocytoma and paraganglioma: A systematic review and individual patient meta-analysis. Endocrine-Related Cancer. 2019;**26**(5):539-550

[46] Al-Sharefi A, Javaid U, Perros P, et al. Clinical presentation and outcomes of phaeochromocytomas/paragangliomas in neurofibromatosis type 1. European Endocrinology. 2019;**15**(2):95-100

[47] Ilanchezhian M, Jha A, Pacak K, Del Rivero J. Emerging treatments for advanced/metastatic pheochromocytoma and paraganglioma. Current Treatment Options in Oncology. 2020;**21**:85

[48] Mak IYF, Hayes A, Khoo B, Grossman A. Peptide receptor radionuclide therapy as a novel treatment for metastatic and invasive Phaeochromocytoma and paraganglioma. Neuroendocrinology. 2019;**109**:287-298

[49] Averbuch SD, Steakley CS, Young RC, et al. Malignant pheochromocytoma: Effective treatment with a combination of cyclophosphamide, vincristine,

and dacarbazine. Annals of Internal Medicine. 1988;**109**(4):267-273

[50] Bechmann N, Moskopp ML, Ullrich M, et al. HIF2α supports pro-metastatic behavior in pheochromocytomas/paragangliomas. Endocrine-Related Cancer. 2020;**27**(11):625-640. DOI: 10.1530/ERC-20-0205

[51] Remacha L, Santos M, et al. Integrative multi-omics analysis identifies a prognostic miRNA signature and a targetable miR-21-3p/TSC2/mTOR axis in metastatic pheochromocytoma/paraganglioma. Theranostics. 2019;**9**:4946-4958. DOI: 10.7150/thno.35458

[52] Nölting S, Grossman A, Pacak K. Metastatic Phaeochromocytoma: Spinning towards more promising treatment options. Experimental and Clinical Endocrinology & Diabetes. 2019;**127**:117-128. DOI: 10.1055/a-0715-1888

[53] Druce MR, Kaltsas GA, Fraenkel M, Gross DJ, Grossman AB. Novel and evolving therapies in the treatment of malignant phaeochromocytoma: Experience with the mTOR inhibitor everolimus (RAD001). Hormone and Metabolic Research. 2009;**41**(9):697-702. DOI: 10.1055/s-0029-1220687

[54] Amar L, Pacak K, Steichen O, Akker SA, Aylwin SJB, Baudin E, et al. International consensus on initial screening and follow-up of asymptomatic SDHx mutation carriers. Nature Review in Endocrinology. 2021;**17**:435-444. DOI: 10.1038/s41574-021-00492-3

[55] Favier J, Amar L, Gimenez-Roqueplo AP. Paraganglioma and phaeochromocytoma: From genetics to personalized medicine. Nature Reviews. Endocrinology. 2015;**11**(2):101-111